Professional Discipline in Nursing, Midwifery and Health Visiting

Professional Discipline in Nursing, Midwifery and Health Visiting

SECOND EDITION

Including
An Exploration of Professional Accountability for Nurses,
Midwives and Health Visitors

REGINALD H. PYNE
OBE, RGN, RFN, FBIM
Assistant Registrar, Standards & Ethics
United Kingdom Central Council
for Nursing, Midwifery and Health Visiting

OXFORD

BLACKWELL SCIENTIFIC PUBLICATIONS

LONDON EDINBURGH BOSTON

MELBOURNE PARIS BERLIN VIENNA

© 1981, 1992 by
Blackwell Scientific Publications
Editorial offices:
Osney Mead, Oxford OX2 0EL
25 John Street, London WC1N 2BL
23 Ainslie Place, Edinburgh EH3 6AJ
3 Cambridge Center, Cambridge,
  Massachusetts 02142, USA
54 University Street, Carlton,
  Victoria 3053, Australia

Other Editorial Offices:
Librairie Arnette SA
2, rue Casimir-Delavigne
75006 Paris
France

Blackwell Wissenschaft-Verlag
Meinekestrasse 4
D-1000 Berlin 15
Germany

Blackwell MZV
Feldgasse 13
A-1238 Wien
Austria

First Edition published 1981
Second Edition published 1992

Set by DP Photosetting, Aylesbury, Bucks
Printed and bound in Great Britain by
Hartnolls, Bodmin, Cornwall

DISTRIBUTORS
Marston Book Services Ltd
PO Box 87
Oxford OX2 0DT
(*Orders*: Tel: 0865 791155
       Fax: 0865 791927
       Telex: 837515)

USA
Blackwell Scientific Publications, Inc.
3 Cambridge Center
Cambridge, MA 02142
(*Orders*: Tel: 800 759-6102)

Canada
Times Mirror Professional Publishing, Ltd
5240 Finch Avenue East
Scarborough, Ontario M15 5A2
(*Orders*: Tel: 416 298-1588)

Australia
Blackwell Scientific Publications
(Australia) Pty Ltd
54 University Street,
Carlton, Victoria 3053
(*Orders*: Tel: 03 347-0300)

British Library
Cataloguing in Publication Data
Pyne, Reginald H.
  Professional discipline in nursing,
  midwifery and health visiting.
    —2nd. ed.
  1. Nurses. Professional behaviour
  I. Title
  610.73069

ISBN 0–632–02975–7

Dedication

To The Vulnerable Public

Contents

Foreword

Dame Audrey Emerton, Chairman of the United Kingdom Central Council for Nursing, Midwifery and Health Visiting

Nothing is more important to a nurse, midwife or health visitor than delivering safe care of a high standard to a patient, mother and baby or a client.

The current legislation that is contained within the Nurses, Midwives and Health Visitors Act 1979 was arrived at following long consultations with the professions and provides the means for the professions to be self-regulating – something which is carefully explained within the chapters of this book. Legislation is not an easy subject to write about in understandable terms but the author Reg Pyne sets out the important landmarks in a very readable style emphasising the importance of Section 2 of the Act with its requirement that standards of training and professional conduct were to be improved.

Many nurses, midwives and health visitors view professional discipline in a negative way and look upon the mechanisms of the professional conduct committee as a means to mete out punishment, failing to appreciate that the mechanisms are designed to protect the vulnerable public to whom this book is dedicated.

The nurses, midwives and health visitors need to understand fully the theory which underpins the professional disciplinary procedure and this is explained in very explicit terms, leaving no doubt at all to the nurse, midwife or health visitor of his/her accountability as a professional whose name appears on the United Kingdom Central Council's register.

Correlating theory and practice is crucial in gaining full understanding. Within the chapters of this book the practice is well set out both in explanation of the procedures within the Nurses, Midwives and Health Visitors Act and the statutory rules, and through a range of casework examples. These in turn serve to illustrate some of the pertinent issues which have featured before the Professional Conduct Committees, and the outcomes. 'Could this happen where you work?' is certainly a question which applies the individual case and makes it all the more readable and meaningful.

The introduction of the Health Committee within the 1979 legislation has provided an alternative to the Professional Conduct hearing when the practitioner's fitness to practise has been impaired by a health problem. The ability to refer a practitioner to the Health Committee at any stage of the procedure up to the final decision being made by the Professional Conduct Committee ensures fairness to the respondent.

Caring for the carer may seem incongruent with the concept of professional discipline but the work of the Nurses' Welfare Service is set out demonstrating the way in which the Service is organised to give assistance to nurses, midwives and health visitors in a time of desperate need on the part of the individual practitioner.

Nurses, midwives and health visitors need to know and understand fully the way in which their profession is regulated. The presentation of facts and information on the subject are set out in a very user friendly style which leads to the reading of this book being a '*must*' for every practitioner.

Preface

In 1980, at the request of Blackwell Scientific Publications, I wrote the first edition of *Professional Discipline in Nursing – Theory and Practice* and had the pleasure of seeing it appear in print the following year. I was unsure at the time that it was appropriate to be writing a book of its type, however, since the professional disciplinary procedures I was to describe in a substantial part of the text would be replaced, as would the statutory body operating them, on the day to be appointed for the Nurses, Midwives and Health Visitors Act 1979 to come fully into operation.

I am grateful to the publishers for persuading me to go ahead and pleased that I was able to help fill a gap in the market that had been identified. I am delighted to have been told by many practitioners how helpful they found that first edition, both for themselves and for the teaching of others. I am flattered by the degree to which the book has been quoted, referenced or recommended in the writings of other people, some known to me, but many not.

Ten years on I have had the pleasure of responding to a further invitation to write this second edition. This time I have felt no uncertainty, first because the first edition has apparently proved helpful, and second because so much has changed in that decade which needs to be made the subject of report and comment.

I make no apology for again reminding readers that the form of statutory regulation of nursing and midwifery that for many years we have taken for granted did not always exist. In Chapter 3 I rehearse some of the history of professional regulation and registration. This is no exercise in nostalgia, but presented as a reminder of how precious our professional inheritance is, how hard it was won, and how great is our responsibility to our professional successors to hand over to them a profession in good order, both aware of and honouring its reasons for existence. My intention in studying the past and reviewing the present is simply to provide lessons which might contribute to improving the future.

In the first two chapters I have endeavoured to explore the concept of profession and of professional responsibility as related to nursing, midwifery and health visiting and to build a solid foundation on which to develop the subsequent chapters.

In Chapter 4 I explain the statutory structure brought about by the Nurses, Midwives and Health Visitors Act 1979 when it came into operation on 1 July 1983, and refer to the challenges and opportunities it brought.

I cannot conceal the excitement I still feel whenever I read Section 2(1) of that Act with its requirement that standards of training and professional conduct were to be improved. The presence of the words *principal*, *shall* and *improve* in a mere 25 word sentence in primary legislation continues to amaze me. In Chapter 5 I elaborate upon some of the measures taken by the United Kingdom Central Council for Nursing, Midwifery and Health Visiting since 1983, commenting particularly on the Code of Professional Conduct and its importance.

Chapters 6, 7 and 8, together with Appendix 1, constitute something of a handbook. Chapter 6 provides a detailed explanation of the system for investigating and judging allegations of misconduct in a professional sense. Chapter 7 explains the entirely new system for considering alleged unfitness to practise due to illness which was made possible by the 1979 Act and which has now operated very successfully for over six years. Both chapters conclude with some statistical information and both link to Appendix 1. Chapter 8 is included to inform the reader about the existence of a specialist social work agency and to explain how it operates to assist practitioners either involved in or at risk of becoming involved in the caseload of the committees described in Chapters 6 and 7. The continued existence of this important service – the Nurses' Welfare Service – influences the work of those committees in a constructive way.

In Chapter 9, using the evidence of the type and quality of cases coming before the Professional Conduct Committee and Health Committee of the UKCC and my own observations, I offer a personal view of the state of the professions when measured against the Code of Professional Conduct and other associated UKCC advisory documents. I also offer some thoughts about the lessons that, in my view, emerge from that same material about managers and employers of nurses, midwives and health visitors.

I devote Chapter 10 to an examination of the law which has operated since July 1983 and offer a personel view of its good points, its bad points, and the way to convert the latter to the former. Chapter 11 is a short concluding statement.

Chapters 12 and 13 provide a number of case studies which can be used by individual practitioners or (supplementing Chapter 6) for group study or seminars with practitioners at all levels.

The studies in Chapter 12 are all based on actual cases which have been the subject of hearings before the UKCC's Professional Conduct Committee in recent years. They are deliberately headed 'Could This Happen Where You Work?' and should be examined with that question in mind and not by way of spending a ghoulish hour looking at other people's misfortunes.

The studies in Chapter 13 are different. They are simply little cameo studies reflecting some of the dilemmas in exercising their accountability that have been shared with me by practitioners. They are offered, in association with Chapters 1, 2, 5 and 9 and Appendices 2 and 3, as a means of exploring this thing called professional accountability.

Appendix 1 reproduces the full text of a UKCC document which has been produced primarily for the benefit of potential complainants but which will clearly prove helpful to many other people both within and outside the professions regulated by the UKCC.

Appendix 2 and Appendix 3 reproduce other UKCC advisory documents which supplement the Code of Professional Conduct, the full text of which can be found in Chapter 5.

The final Appendix (4) provides 'answers' in that it indicates what decisions the Professional Conduct Committee made on the cases in Chapter 12 and comments on the 'Aspects of Accountability' studies in Chapter 13.

For the entire period since the Nurses, Midwives and Health Visitors Act 1979 came into operation I have been privileged to be a member of the staff of the United Kingdom Central Council for Nursing, Midwifery and Health Visiting, for much of the time as its Director for Professional Conduct and more recently as Assistant Registrar for Standards and Ethics. I emphasise, however, that while the views that I express in this book have been developed while I have held those posts they are my own views and not necessarily those of the Council.

I hope and trust that this book will stimulate many practitioners to explore for themselves the concept of profession, the implications of professional accountability and the importance of professional self-regulation.

Reginald Pyne
January 1991

Acknowledgements

It has been my privilege to prepare a new edition of *Professional Discipline in Nursing* and to widen the subject matter covered. I am grateful to Blackwell Scientific Publications, and in particular Ann Morris and Richard Miles for persuading me to do it.

I acknowledge my gratitude to my professional colleagues on the staff of the United Kingdom Central Council for Nursing, Midwifery and Health Visiting whose stimulating company and conversation assists in the formation of views that eventually emerge in published form.

I am grateful to the Council for permission to reproduce four of its documents which have an obvious relevance to the subject of this book and for the privilege that has been mine of working as one of its senior professional staff during a period of exciting challenge, change and professional development.

I acknowledge my gratitude to the staff of the Professional Conduct Division of the Council with whom it was my privilege to work for a number of years before transferring to my present role.

I acknowledge my gratitude for the friendship and support of those who have served as members of the UKCC for any period of time since it was brought into existence by the Nurses, Midwives and Health Visitors Act 1979.

Last, but certainly not least, I acknowledge the support of both my excellent personal assistant, Christine Simmons and my wife, Maureen who have converted my badly written manuscript into the attractively typed document I have been able to deliver to my publishers.

Chapter 1

What is a Profession?

What is a profession? What does membership of a profession involve? What exactly is professional accountability? Can the separate yet substantially interlinked occupational groups called nurses, midwives and health visitors honestly claim to constitute professions? These questions are often posed by people with enquiring minds, many of them practitioners within these groups. The answers they receive are not always adequate. I believe that nursing, midwifery and health visiting can justly claim to constitute a profession or a linked set of professions for reasons that I trust will become clear as the pages of this book are turned.

As for the other questions, after a decade of employment in a post which required me to operate the system whereby the profession of nursing in England and Wales was to some extent regulated through the statutory body's disciplinary process, and much of another decade fulfilling a similar function in respect of nurses, midwives and health visitors in the United Kingdom, I hold to the conclusion that consideration of some negative aspects (e.g. professional misconduct, professional negligence, professional irresponsibility) often helps to provide clues to some satisfactory answers. Let me illustrate what I mean.

A young woman appeared before the Professional Conduct Committee only a year after she first registered following successful completion of her training programme. This followed her appearance in a magistrates court where she had pleaded guilty to the theft of drugs and unlawful possession of drugs. She had been dealt with sympathetically by the magistrates, being given a conditional discharge for 12 months. She was the epitome of the person you would never expect to see in this situation.

The story began some months earlier when this young woman returned from a holiday in sunny climes with some friends. It had apparently been one of those energetic holidays which leaves you, on your return, in need of another holiday to recover. She returned to her hospital work, looking visibly tired. On only her second day back she was approached by one of the hospital porters. He was well known for his friendly and jocular remarks to everybody, irrespective of status and position, so she was neither surprised or offended when he smilingly commented on her tired appearance. She simply explained that it was all the product of her good holiday which had left little time for sleep.

The friendly porter offered her a tablet which he said would 'pick her up'. Unwisely she accepted it. It was an amphetamine tablet. Some days later events took a more sinister turn. The nurse was again approached by the same man, but now the mood was not at all friendly! He reminded her of the unprescribed tablet she had freely accepted from him. He reminded her that, as a qualified nurse, she knew better than to have done so and he could now get her into a great deal of trouble. He promised not to do so, however, provided she obtained more drugs for him from the ward on which she was working.

In a state of great anxiety and fear, she did exactly that for several days, obtaining tranquillisers and sedatives by forging prescriptions.

After several days she came to her senses and realised that each further such action simply pushed her deeper into trouble. She lived at home and enjoyed a good relationship with her mother. She told her mother exactly what was happening and asked her to go with her to the police and subsequently to her nurse manager. As a result of her confession the police were able to detain the porter and obtain convictions for numerous offences concerning obtaining and supplying a substantial range of drugs.

While the magistrates who heard the case saw the event as uncharacteristic and took a lenient view, the employers decided to dismiss her. There had been nothing in her previous record as a student nurse in the same location, or as a staff nurse to suggest that her conduct had been anything other than satisfactory, but she was guilty of a serious breach of trust and abuse of her professional position.

The Professional Conduct Committee now had to decide whether this offence and the nurse's retrospective view of it were such that members of the public, when at their most vulnerable, were safe in her hands.

This case says a number of things that might assist in providing answers to some of the questions in the opening paragraph of this chapter. It illustrates that nurses, midwives and health visitors are subject to the law of the land in the same way as all other citizens. It then goes further and illustrates that nurses, midwives and health visitors who offend in such a manner will also be the subject of consideration and judgment by certain of their professional peers who, acting on behalf of the profession as a whole, have to consider their appropriateness to continue as members of the profession with all its privileges and responsibilities. In this case, while in no way condoning the unwise, illegal and unprofessional actions of the nurse, the Committee took the view that it was uncharacteristic, that she had derived substantial lessons from the whole sad experience and that there seemed to be no prospect of any repetition of this or other unprofessional actions. The information received about her knowledge, skill and competence as a nurse was impressive. The Committee decided that her name should not be removed from the register for the misconduct proved in a public hearing, but that some words of caution and counsel would suffice.

The matters raised in that case may be taken a step further by consideration of another case.

One day a consultant anaesthetist whose work took him to the operating department of a small hospital only one day each week, when about to sign for the administration of a drug in the controlled drug register, observed some entries which purported to be his and spontaneously declared that somebody had been forging his signature.

In the course of the enquiry that ensued a theatre sister admitted that she had misappropriated two 100 mg ampoules of pethidine from the theatre stock and made fictitious and forged entries in the register to cover their removal. Possessed of her written admission, her professional managers dismissed her from employment and reported the matter to the police. The police decided not to prosecute because the monetary value of the drugs did not reach the arbitrary level they were imposing at the time, below which they would not prosecute for theft.

The nurse appealed against dismissal from employment. Her appeal was heard by three members of the district health authority who upheld her appeal and ordered her re-instatement on the basis that the police had not instituted criminal proceedings. Her admission had not been retracted.

Faced with this situation, and mindful of her own wider professional responsibilities, the senior nurse suspended the nurse on full salary, but also reported the case to the statutory body for investigation and judgment. In due course the nurse admitted the facts at a Professional Conduct Committee. Those facts were adjudged to be misconduct. After hearing of the nurse's previous record and what she had to offer in mitigation the Committee determined to remove her name from the professional register.

This case also makes a number of useful points. It illustrates that an employer's decision about a person's employment status is purely incidental to the regulatory body's decision about his or her status as a registered nurse. The same would be true if the decision to uphold an appeal had been that of an industrial tribunal or employment appeal tribunal. Further to that, it illustrates that nurse managers, faced with a situation of that kind, have a judgment to make. They cannot simply abrogate their personal professional responsibility on the basis of a possibly arbitrary or unwise decision made by other people. It also indicates that the statutory bodies charged with the responsibility to determine, for the professions they regulate, what, in a particular set of circumstances, is misconduct in a professional sense are not dependent on the criminal courts to establish guilt. They can receive allegations direct and, having operated the procedures which the law prescribes, arrive at appropriate conclusions.

Let us consider just one more case before turning again to the original series of questions.

At the conclusion of a hearing in which the charge against him had been proved on the evidence of several witnesses and then been regarded as misconduct in a professional sense, a psychiatric unit charge nurse was removed from the register by the Professional Conduct Committee. The very professional charge against him was that of '. . . failing to give appropriate care to a patient in his charge' in a number of specified respects.

He subsequently exercised his right of appeal to the appeal court, as a result of which the case became the subject of review by two judges.

This third case is cited not because the presiding appeal judge and his fellow judge dismissed the appeal, but because in doing so they emphasised that their primary role in considering such a case was to examine the evidence as to fact that had been given and decide whether a reasonable group of people, assembled as the Professional Conduct Committee, faced with that evidence, could find the allegations proved to the required standard. That standard, like that applying in criminal courts, is that the Committee must be satisfied so that it is sure – satisfied beyond reasonable doubt. The judges, having determined that the evidence had established the facts, indicated that they saw it as no part of their role to question the decision of a specialist committee, composed primarily of practising nurses, who had resolved that the facts did constitute misconduct in a professional sense and that removal from the register was the appropriate judgment in the public interest.

So even the eminent judges who sit in the Royal Courts of Justice accept that the nursing, midwifery and health visiting professions, through the statutory framework established by Parliament, have been given the authority to regulate themselves in the public interest and therefore have to make their own decisions as to the kind of conduct that warrants removal from a practitioner of the right to practise.

Now let us look again at the questions that opened this chapter: What is a profession? What does membership of a profession involve? What is professional accountability? Can nursing, midwifery and health visiting honestly claim to be a profession or a group of related professions?

Dictionaries are an obvious source of definitions, but sadly, in respect of any attempt to grasp the concept of 'profession' they are far from adequate. The word is more often defined as relating to the vows of a religious community than to any specialist areas of employment. Similarly the word *professional* seems, in the way it is defined in dictionaries, to have more to do with participating in sport for gain than with membership of an occupational group composed of people who recognise and adhere to certain ethical standards. This is not to say, however, that a study of several dictionaries is a wasted exercise. The following phrases have been extracted from the definitions of the word *profession*:

'A calling requiring specialised knowledge and often long, intensive academic preparation.' (*Webster's New Collegiate Dictionary*, 1980)   [1]

'A vocation in which a professed knowledge of some department of learning is used in its application to the affairs of others, or in the practise of an art founded upon it.' (*The Shorter Oxford English Dictionary*, 1973)   [2]

'Occupation requiring training and intellectual abilities, practised so as to earn a living.' (*The Penguin English Dictionary*, 1965)   [3]

'An employment, not mechanical, and requiring some degree of learning.' (*Chambers Twentieth Century Dictionary*, 1972)   [4]

'An occupation, especially one that involves knowledge and training in a branch of advanced learning.' (*The Oxford Paperback Dictionary*, 1979)   [5]

These definitions at least have the merit of containing some relevant words and phrases, such as *learning, knowledge, academic preparation, training* and *an art founded on knowledge*. If, like me, you still find them woefully inadequate as you seek to apply them to the art and science of nursing, midwifery and health visiting, I suggest you note that they would prove equally inadequate when applied to the other regulated health professions. One might expect that a study of the definitions of *professionalism* would prove helpful. It does not, because it constantly relates back to what (for my present purposes) are the inadequate or unsatisfactory definitions of *profession* set before you.

So where else can we turn for assistance as we attempt to grasp and understand the concept of *profession* and to provide criteria against which to measure those occupational groups called nurses, midwives and health visitors? There may be other sources to which we could turn but my preferred published statement is (perhaps surprisingly) one that appeared in the 'Letters to the Editor' columns of the *Daily Telegraph* in 1978. The writer of the letter (J. Ralph

Blanchfield) first commented on the tendency to misuse and abuse the word *profession* and the need to define it, and then continued:

'Profession' cannot be defined in terms of any single characteristic. To justify the description, an occupational group must fulfil not some but all of the following criteria:

1. Its practice is based on a recognised body of learning.
2. It establishes an independent body for the collective pursuit of aims and objects related to these criteria.
3. Admission to corporate membership is based on strict standards of competence attested by examinations and assessed experience.
4. It recognises that its practice must be for the benefit of the public as well as that of its practitioners.
5. It recognises its responsibility to advance and extend the body of knowledge on which it is based.
6. It recognises its responsibility to concern itself with facilities, methods and provision for educating and training future entrants and for enhancing the knowledge of present practitioners.
7. It recognises the need for its members to conform to high standards of ethics and professional conduct set out in a published code with appropriate disciplinary procedures.

Does this improve on the definitions drawn from a selection of dictionaries? I believe the answer is an unequivocal 'Yes'. Those dictionaries variously described the role as calling, vocation, occupation and employment. They also refer variously to the specialised knowledge, academic preparation, department of learning, training and knowledge on which it is based. In this respect they compare only with the first of the seven points in the Blanchfield definition. Ironically it is on this very point that some people argue that nursing is not a profession. Nursing (they say) cannot be regarded as a profession because it is based not on a body of knowledge of its own but that of the medical profession.

Whilst I readily accept that much of the role of the nurse (and, to a substantial degree, the midwife) is concerned with the administration of medicines and the provision of treatment prescribed by doctors, there is very much more to nursing, midwifery and health visiting than that. I have no doubt that many patients who received, from nurses and midwives, only the treatment prescribed by doctors would feel very aggrieved. The many other things that go to make nursing, midwifery and health visiting practice what it is are based on an existing and continually developing body of knowledge and practical skills which, while often (not always) applied as a complement to prescribed medical treatment and drugs, can stand and often do stand on their own. On this knowledge and these skills those who aspire to achieve qualifications as registered nurses, midwives or health visitors are examined and assessed. It is therefore my contention that the three linked professions of which I write do satisfy the first criterion of the Blanchfield definition.

What of the other criteria? The second is clearly satisfied by the existence, as required by the Nurses, Midwives and Health Visitors Act 1979, of the statutory body called the United Kingdom Central Council for Nursing, Midwifery and Health Visiting (UKCC or the Council). That Act places upon the regulatory body which it has created not simply aims and objectives but the mandatory requirement that standards of training and professional conduct shall be established and improved. I explore the response to this challenge in a later chapter.

The third criterion is satisfied in several ways. As required by the Nurses, Midwives and Health Visitors Act 1979, subordinate legislation (rules set out in statutory instruments), prepared by the UKCC, state the requirements to be satisfied and the competences to be achieved for admission to the register as a nurse, midwife or health visitor. The UKCC also prescribes the kind, content and standard of training required. Applicants for admission to the register in the United Kingdom following initial training and registration in other countries (excluding those from the European Community covered by specialist directives who have freedom of movement within the Community) are subjected to individual evaluation.

The fourth criterion – recognition by an occupational group that its practice must be for the benefit of the public – has effectively been answered in law, even if not explicitly stated therein, since the first Midwives Act 1902 and the Nurses Registration Act 1919. It has become more overt through the wording of the Nurses, Midwives and Health Visitors Act 1979[6] and is stated in bold and clear terms in documents prepared and issued by the new regulatory body established by that Act since it succeeded to the role of the replaced bodies, and took on a much wider regulatory role in July 1983.

It is probably true to say of the fifth criterion that, while always receiving some attention, this area had perhaps received less attention than it needed and deserved. This is no longer the case. The number of practitioners engaged in valid research is most impressive. The much larger number voluntarily engaging in work directed to identifying ways in which standards of care can be improved and then establishing the means of achieving the new standards is greater still. In both respects this is extremely encouraging.

As for criterion 6, both from the profession's statutory body (UKCC) through its statements of its expectations of practitioners on its register, and from those practitioners as they work out their individual ways of responding through their practice and in their various practice settings, comes a clear indication that this responsibility is understood and accepted.

The final criterion in the Blanchfield definition requires that an occupational group '. . . recognises the need for its members to conform to high standards of professional conduct set out in a published code with appropriate disciplinary procedures'. Nursing, midwifery and health visiting undoubtedly satisfy this requirement, as the remainder of this book asserts and Chapters 5 and 6 illustrate.

I will assert, then, that, measured against the most satisfactory definition of a profession that I have been able to find, nursing, midwifery and health visiting justify that description and title. That does not, however, mean that I believe that definition to be perfect. There is one particular respect in which I would dispute the wording to some degree, though recognising that the differences are more of a semantic nature than of principles. It relates to the fourth criterion in the list. For me, one of the hallmarks of a profession is that it accepts the onerous burden of regulating itself, but recognises that this is to be performed for the protection of the public and not the prestige of its members. Such an arrangement exists for nursing, midwifery and health visiting in the United Kingdom. It is something precious which the members of the profession must safeguard.

I hope that I have satisfactorily answered two of the questions with which I opened this chapter – 'What is a profession?' and 'Can the occupational groups called nurses, midwives and health visitors claim to constitute professions?' What of the remaining two? One asks 'What does membership of a profession involve?' and the other 'What exactly is professional accountability?' On reflection I think that these questions identify two facets of the same point – that which will form the subject of Chapter 5. For now I content myself with simply stating in broad terms that any person on the Council's register – nurse, midwife or health visitor – irrespective of the post he or she holds, bears a personal professional accountability which cannot be avoided in four specific areas. These I believe to be:

(1) his or her own standards of care and the knowledge, skill, attitudes, values and qualities of observation on which they are based;
(2) his or her concern about the environment in which he or she has to practise;
(3) his or her responsibility to care for and about colleagues; and
(4) his or her acceptance of a role that includes participation in the teaching of others, be they patients, clients, students or junior colleagues.

To those who accept posts which have a managerial component falls that additional burden (shared, with enthusiasm I hope, by those with line management responsibility) of striving, at all times, to create, sustain and maintain a setting and approach which is dynamic, so that all nurses, midwives and health visitors (not only those in training) may grow and improve, and thus contribute to growth and improvement in others. This duty, like the four listed above, is concerned with the safety of patients and clients and the standards of care available for them now and in the future.

These then are, in my view, some of the key points to make in respect of those remaining questions. You may not necessarily agree with them. Whether you do ot not at this stage, I suggest that you defer judgment until you have read Chapter 5. I respect your right then to come to different conclusions about those things that constitute professional accountability and illustrate what membership of a profession involves. If my conclusions do not appeal to you I suggest that you prepare a list of your own.

I have little doubt that if you do that it will lead you, as it has me, to the conclusion that the nursing, midwifery and health visiting profession, through each and every one of its members must come to a recognition of its collective responsibility for regulating itself. While a special and substantial part of that responsibility is laid by the law of the country on the United Kingdom Central Council for Nursing, Midwifery and Health Visiting (through its power in respect of individuals and institutions), the remaining part, and undoubtedly the largest part, must come from the self-discipline of the profession's members. Without that, no matter how we define their word *profession*, we shall not deserve that honoured title.

(Chapter 12 provides further case studies concerning Professional Conduct Committee work and relates to the contents of Chapter 6, for individual or group consideration.)

(Chapter 13 provides case studies concerning the exercise of accountability related to the contents of Chapter 5.)

REFERENCES

[1] *Webster's New Collegiate Dictionary*, Eighth Edition (1980). Springfield, Mass.: G. & C. Merriam Co. By permission. From *Webster's New Collegiate Dictionary* © 1980 by G. & C. Merriam Co., Publishers of the Merriam-Webster Dictionaries.

[2] The Shorter Oxford English Dictionary, Third Edition (1973). Edited by C.T. Onions. Oxford: Oxford University Press. Excerpts reprinted by permission of Oxford University Press.

[3] *The Penguin English Dictionary* (1969). Edited by G. N. Garmonsay & J. Simpson. Harmondsworth: Penguin Books. Reprinted by permission of Penguin Books.

[4] *Chambers Twentieth Century Dictionary* (1972). Edited by A.M. Macdonald. Edinburgh & London: W. & R. Chambers Ltd.

[5] *The Oxford Paperback Dictionary* (1969). Edited by J.M. Hawkins. Oxford: Oxford University Press. Excerpt reprinted by permission of Oxford University Press.

[6] *Nurses, Midwives & Health Visitors Act 1979.* London: HMSO.

Chapter 2

The Concept of Professional Discipline

The previous chapter concluded with reference to the profession's responsibility for regulating itself and the importance within that activity of the self-discipline of its members. This chapter seeks to explore the concept of professional discipline that was touched upon in the closing words.

What is professional discipline? Is it concerned with professional ethics or conduct or standards of practice? Possibly these questions, as with those asked at the beginning of Chapter 1, may be best approached by considering first a negative aspect of the subject. I do not mean that we should, at this stage, consider the consequences of a lack of discipline on the part of members of the nursing, midwifery, and health visiting professions: the concerns I have about that lack and the evidence on which those concerns are based will emerge in subsequent chapters. The negative aspect that I have in mind is rather that as we educate aspiring practitioners in the theory and practice of the profession and as we introduce them to the role that they must fulfil as qualified professional practitioners, we so often fail to develop in them an understanding of what professional accountability means.

This conclusion was well illustrated by the case of a psychiatric nurse who appeared before the Professional Conduct Committee of the UKCC to answer charges alleging misconduct resulting from his conviction in a criminal court of cultivating cannabis plants at his home and possessing a quantity of medicines that were the property of his health authority employer. (The medicines were mild analgesics, expectorants and vitamins.) When asked by a member of the committee that was to decide whether he should retain or lose the right to practise how he viewed the matter in retrospect he, like so many others, gave an answer which was based only on the effect it had on him and his life. There was no evident appreciation of the significance of his contravention of the law, his casual self-medication or of the damage to the public's trust in the profession that might have resulted from the publicity about his court appearance. He simply said that he was foolish, because he had lost a good job that was convenient to his home and with quite good pay.

Another case which illustrates the same failure to understand what professional accountability means and involves, featured a registered general nurse employed as charge nurse in a large general hospital. He also had appeared in a criminal court and been convicted, on his own plea of guilty, of dishonestly obtaining a quantity of Brufen tablets on two occasions, these being the property of his health authority employer. It emerged that he had a friend who suffered from arthritis, for which Brufen had been regularly prescribed. On two occasions that friend, having failed to obtain a further prescription in time, found his supply exhausted and asked the nurse (who became the respondent in the case) to obtain some tablets for him. He readily acquiesced. To obtain a supply he made out a patient's treatment chart for a fictional patient and signed it himself, forging a doctor's signature. The matter came to light when, having obtained a second supply in the same way, he was careless enough to leave the fictitious treatment chart on the office desk where it was found by the doctor whose forged signature it bore.

When you have considered Chapter 6 and Appendix 1 you might care to consider, how, had you been a member of the Professional Conduct Committee, you would have chosen to conclude these two cases.

Would you regard the nurses who were the subject of these cases as guilty of indiscipline, irresponsibility or a failure to honour their accountability? Are these, perhaps, the same thing? There may be some merit in turning again to the same dictionaries (accessed for the purposes of Chapter 1) to assist in arriving at some definition of our terms.

DISCIPLINE

First, *discipline*. Unfortunately those dictionaries prove no more helpful with this word than they did with the word *profession*. I say this because, where the word is used as a noun, it tends for the most part to be identified with other words and phrases that do not really approach the interpretation that members of recognised professions would seek. For example, the word is variously identified as 'instruction', 'order', 'mortification', 'punishment', 'training that moulds the mental faculties', 'training in the practice of arms' and others in similar vein. While I accept that all these words and phrases are valid in defining *discipline*, they do not satisfy my requirements as I seek for an explanation of 'professional discipline'.

Buried within the larger definitions, however, there are some points that do help, even if they are not entirely satisfactory. For instance, 'mode of life in accordance with rules', 'orderly or prescribed pattern of behaviour', 'a rule or system of rules governing conduct or activity', 'a system of rules for conduct' and 'self-control'.

In spite of the fact that some of these definitions seem to describe some controlling features of nursing from which it has been necessarily striving to break free, that does, I suggest, take us forward at least a little. If, at this stage, I have to particularise as to why I am not entirely satisfied I would state that it is because of the emphasis on 'rules'. In respect of any occupational or vocational group which can rightly claim the name *profession* I maintain that the rules are concerned with the structure within which the profession is managed and operates and should not be used to define acceptable and unacceptable behaviour. What is acceptable or unacceptable behaviour has to be decided by considering it in its context.

PROFESSIONAL MISCONDUCT

With the passing of each year of my direct involvement with the profession's disciplinary machinery I have become more convinced that to respond to the pressures that are often applied to define professional misconduct by producing a list of proscribed actions would be dangerous, since the circumstances in which incidents raise the question 'Is this misconduct in a professional sense?' are rarely the same. For example, although in the vast majority of situations it would be quite wrong to disclose information received from a patient in confidence, there are rare and exceptional circumstances in which it would be right to do so. Therefore to ensure in statutory rules a list of actions and omissions that are considered misconduct would be bad both for members of the profession and members of the public.

It would be unsatisfactory and unjust for members of the profession if the context of an alleged offence (often unreasonable by virtue of excessive pressure of work, unclear policies, inadequate management, etc.) were not to be considered before labelling an episode of behaviour 'professional misconduct'. For the public who depend upon the availability of a competent and caring service from persons on the UKCC's register, it would also be unsatisfactory because no list prepared now could possibly cater for all the eventualities in as little as five years' time. Could our predecessors have possibly contemplated the need to include in such a list attempts to unreasonably resist patients' access to their records, for example? I doubt it very much. The inevitable conclusion drawn by those faced with the task of producing such a list would be that it had to be produced in such general terms that it would be better to have no such document at all. Besides, would such a closely defined set of rules on 'misconduct' (even if it could be kept up to date, which is unlikely in the extreme) be consistent with membership of a profession whose practitioners must be constantly engaged in the exercise of personal judgment, and in an often imperfect environment?

RESPONSIBILITY

Now to the word *responsibility*. Here I find my dictionaries more to my liking, since they clearly indicate (a) that to be responsible is to be obliged, either legally or morally, to take care of something or to carry out a duty, and (b) that one is liable to be blamed for failure. Surely these are things about which nurses, midwives and health visitors know a great deal and which they accept as a necessary consequence of their professional status.

Lack of responsibility, however, is not something that is manifested only by practitioners in direct clinical practice. Those who have accepted the different responsibility associated with nursing, midwifery or health visiting managerial positions often reveal it just as strongly. When that happens the consequences may be still more serious, because the manager who fails to act responsibly not only affects for ill the service to patients or clients but creates a situation in which his or her own staff may be put at risk. The consequences may be made heavier still if a decision is made which seeks a short-term solution to the problem with no thought for the long-term consequences.

One case heard by the Professional Conduct Committee which illustrates this phenomenon involved a 33-year-old registered general nurse who had been employed as the senior sister in an intensive therapy unit. She had been found staggering about in the unit early one afternoon and, when asked what was wrong by a colleague, said that she had ingested two or three sodium amytal tablets from a bottle which had been in the possession of a patient admitted earlier that day. On the face of it this appeared to be a serious offence on the part of the sister. The evidence of the background to the incident, however, revealed her as more victim than villain.

It emerged that, some months earlier, the nursing officer to whom this sister had line responsibility had to be admitted to hospital for a planned major operation. It was known that she would be absent for several months. It was also known that no cover for her duties could be organised. The more senior nurse manager admitted that they took stock of their position. They agreed that this sister was totally reliable and that they need not worry themselves about that unit, instead concentrating their stretched management resources in those areas where the sisters were, in their view, less reliable or experienced.

The sister's normal link to more senior management had gone. In no time at all the pressure on her increased as the unit became progressively more busy, there was severe staff shortage, little continuity, and the staff she had were often of inadequate quality or experience. Being the kind of person she was – highly skilled and committed – the sister waited for her managers to notice her dilemma rather than telling them. So she began and continued to work quite excessive hours to keep the unit going and stopped leaving the unit for meal breaks. Nobody seemed to notice the stress to which she was subject or how terribly tired she was.

On the day of the incident, once again she did not leave the unit for lunch, but simply snatched a few minutes for a cup of coffee in the staff room. It was then that she swallowed the tablets which (inevitably in her tired condition) acted very quickly. She tried to return to her duties but her condition led a colleague to call a senior nurse manager. Then that manager became aware of just how great were the burdens this sister had been bearing – so great that when they removed her they had to close the unit.

Once the full picture had been seen and understood the immediate managers were kind and helpful. They channelled the sister to appropriate medical help and reassured her about her future employment. They also involved the support of the Nurses Welfare Service about which you can read in Chapter 8. Her appearance before the Professional Conduct Committee resulted from a complaint by a more senior manager.

That case illustrates the type of problem that can develop for a practitioner who is too compliant, too submissive and lacking in assertiveness. It also illustrates that management is not simply about waiting to be told about the problems but walking the job so that they are identified. It can be recorded that the immediate managers in this case recognised their failure and learnt from the experience. It is not always so, as the following example illustrates.

A 28-year-old registered general nurse became the subject of a Professional Conduct Committee hearing following a conviction in a magistrates court for theft of a considerable quantity of pethidine, fortral, syringes and needles from the company for which she worked as an occupational health nurse. A psychiatrist's report, submitted to the committee in evidence, revealed that a year earlier, when employed as a ward sister, she had been discovered misappropriating diazepam from her ward stock. She had (the report indicated) been quietly asked to resign, in return for which the nurse managers would take no further action on the matter. She did resign and quickly found employment with the heavy engineering company where controlled drugs were (of necessity) stocked and the control system (regrettably) was almost non-existent. The consequences you have been told.

This was a case in which the nurse concerned was not the only one who failed to act responsibly. Those nurse managers also have much to answer for since, in seeking a short-term solution to their immediate problem and thus succeeding in their desire to avoid any bad publicity for 'their hospital', they abrogated most aspects of their professional responsibility. In disposing of this nurse from their employment but doing nother further either to channel her to help or to question her continued appropriateness to be a registered nurse they were simply (to put the best possible interpretation on it) acting to protect their particular patients at that time. Meanwhile, however, they were neglecting their responsibilities to their profession and its standards and they were neglecting their responsibilities for this possibly sick colleague. By their failure the public were put at risk and this colleague was allowed to progress further into drug dependence, then requiring more time and much more medical and social work help to achieve her rehabilitation.

After reading Chapter 5 you might care to analyse the behaviour of all the participants in the cases described above. One of the lessons to emerge is certainly that while professional nurses, midwives and health visitors are accountable for their own actions, and while those practitioners who take up managerial posts bear special responsibilities which relate both to the public and to members of the profession, all members of the profession have responsibility to care for and about each other.

Unfortunately, although there is evidence that it has been changing for the better in recent years, it seems that there are still too many practitioners who choose to look the other way or not to interfere when they suspect or know that a colleague is behaving unprofessionally. Quite apart from the fact that this allows that colleague to go on putting herself at risk, it places patients at risk from a possibly unsafe practitioner. Some registered practitioners, by their unquestioning response to certain requests and by their willingness to disregard carefully prepared policies, so often unwittingly fail their colleagues, their profession and (most of all) their patients and clients. Just one more illustration must suffice.

A staff nurse on night duty in a large city general hospital expressed concern that another nurse was 'borrowing' pethidine from her ward very often, and suggested to the night sister that the ward in question ought to organise itself better so that the night staff did not need to 'borrow' a drug that was in frequent use. This innocent report led to an investigation which, revealed that another registered nurse had been obtaining pethidine not only from that ward but also from many other wards in this large hospital. Still more, it revealed that the 'borrowing' was taking place when the ward's stock was more than adequate to respond to the current prescriptions. This very large amount of pethidine (on average 700 mg each night shift worked over several months) was illegally and fraudulently obtained by the nurse by the simple expedient of going to other wards with treatment cards of fictitious patients and stating 'I have to give this patient some pethidine and I have run out. Can I borrow some?' In ward after ward, other registered nurses were providing the pethidine, recording its administration in their ward drug recording book and signing as having witnessed the administration when all they had witnessed was another nurse leaving the ward with an ampoule and a treatment card for a non-existent patient. And all this in a hospital which had a good, specific and easily available policy concerning the administration of medicines. So much for personal responsibility for one's actions.

CONCLUSION

So what is professional discipline? Surely it is two things. At the individual level

I believe it to be the self-discipline of the members of the profession – their individual determination to act in a responsible way and in accordance with the moral principles of their profession. At the collective level I see it as the process by which the professions of nursing, midwifery and health visiting (acting not in their own interest but on behalf of the public) operate that section of the law that permits the application of appropriate sanctions to its culpable members impaired by illness.

Sir David Napley, in an address to the veterinary profession in 1987, said:

'The characteristic most resented by those who attack the professions – our independence – is the very characteristic of a true profession and that which provides the greatest measure of protection for the public. Independence means an exemption from external control or support.'[1]

To that Joy Wingfield has added:

'Independence also implies a voluntary submission by the professional to control and review of his behaviour by his peers.

Although this control must be exercised in a fair and judicial manner, self-discipline is infinitely more demanding than the basic levels of morality established at law.'[2]

Professional discipline is inextricably entwined with the whole theme of responsibility. This is one of eight key words around which Baroness Macfarlane built an article in 1980 as she expressed her hopes for nursing in the decade then to come. That decade has now passed, but the words remain valid and applicable to another decade. In that article it was stated that:

'We also have a responsibility for our own professional actions. This is legally a fact, but as professionals we make decisions about the nursing care of individuals and we must be seen to be accountable for the clinical decisions we make and the actions we carry out. A developing sense of professional responsibility and accountability for clinical nursing actions by the practising nurse are priorities as we enter the next decade.'[3]

I was delighted when that article was first published to read such a positive statement, since we so often think and speak in negative terms when the subject is 'discipline' or 'responsibility'. To be self-disciplined and to act responsibly are positive virtues, since without them all the knowledge and skill we possess will consistently fail to provide care of a high standard.

Looking back, I also find it significant that Baroness Macfarlane wrote of '. . . being seen to be accountable . . .' and of '. . . accountability for clinical nursing actions. . .'. Those words 'accountable' and 'accountability' have been the subject of a great deal of exploration and elaboration in recent years. The basis of that interest is a feature of Chapter 5.

REFERENCES

[1] Sir David Napley. *Veterinary Record*, 1987; **121**, 281.
[2] Joy Wingfield. Misconduct and the pharmacist. *The Pharmaceutical Journal*, 27 October 1990.
[3] Baroness Macfarlane. *Nursing Mirror*, 10 January 1980.

Chapter 3

Registration and Regulation: Its Origins and Development

Statutory control of nursing, midwifery and health visiting education and practice has not always existed in the form we know it today. The Nurses, Midwives and Health Visitors Act, which Parliament approved and which received the Royal Assent in 1979, became fully operative on 1 July 1983. On that date an entirely new structure came into existence and operation, with new bodies completely replacing old. Significantly, however, the new registration and regulatory body is possessed of important new powers which are the subject of Chapters 4, 5 and 7.

ORIGINS

Before proceeding to consideration of the new legislation there is merit in taking a brief look back. This is not suggested as an exercise in nostalgia, but as one way of remembering just how precious our professional inheritance is and how great is our responsibility to the future. It is now well over 100 years since the fight for the registration of nurses and midwives seriously began, yet it is easy to observe the various ways in which the concept of 'profession' is still under attack: time indeed to consider the past in order to value the present and prepare for the future.

In 1874, Miss Florence Lees published her book entitled *A Handbook for Ward Sisters*. For the purpose of this chapter, that book is significant because of three short sentences in the preface by Dr (later Sir) Henry Acland, rather than for its main contents. Dr Acland wrote:

> The Medical Act of 1858 allows women to be registered as medical practitioners. It makes no provision for the registration of trained nurses. That this ought to be remedied can hardly admit of doubt.

Even though he was President of the General Medical Council when the book was published, his view that '. . . it can hardly admit of doubt . . .' was not shared by all within his own profession or, indeed, by all nurses. Many immediately expressed their reservations. Doubts surfaced in plenty and, over the years that followed – particularly during the period 1880 to 1900 – the opposing factions furiously debated their various views. The events of this period as they apply to both nursing and midwifery are dealt with at length in two chapters in *Nursing and Midwifery since 1900* (edited by Allan and Jolley).[1] For the present purposes of this chapter it must suffice to state that the first 'Midwives Act' reached the statute book in 1902 and (after some delay because the House of Commons took excessive time on the Dogs Protection Bill) the Nurses Registration Acts,

15

applying the registration and regulation principles to the countries of the United Kingdom, followed in 1919. Formal registration of Health Visitors came only with the Nurses, Midwives and Health Visitors Act 1979, operative from 1983.

The fascinating details of those years and of the traumatic early life of the General Nursing Council for England and Wales are described in the books listed at the end of this chapter to which the enthusiastic student of legislation or nursing and midwifery history can refer.[2,3,4] It is a matter of record, however, that one of the responsibilities placed upon the now replaced statutory bodies by those 1902 and 1919 Acts of Parliament, and which continues to be placed with the United Kingdom Central Council for Nursing, Midwifery and Health Visiting by the Nursing, Midwives and Health Visitors Act of 1979 is that aspect of professional regulation known as professional discipline.

It can be seen, therefore, that from the time when the law first introduced a new regime for training, examination and approval of training institutions, it also required the same bodies it established to undertake not only that work in the public interest but also to exercise a professional disciplinary function. Peer judgment had arrived as an aspect of the law. If a nurse was a subject of complaint which called into question her nurse registration status, it would be primarily nurses who would hear the evidence and decide whether her right to practise should be removed. From the outset the statutory bodies (i.e. the General Nursing Councils and Central Midwives Boards) exercised this important function for the protection of the public, not for the self-aggrandisement of their respective professions.

The new legislation replaced five bodies which had exercised the disciplinary function for one professional group, one country or both profession and country. In my brief retrospective study I use, for illustrative purposes, the former General Nursing Council for England and Wales.

At first, and indeed for many years, all cases were first considered by the Disciplinary and Penal Cases Committee, the members of which had to decide whether a *prima facie* case of misconduct had been established. Where the decision was in the affirmative the case was then considered at a full Council meeting to determine whether or not to remove the practitioner from the register. The disadvantage of this system is clear in retrospect. When a case was forwarded for a hearing, those members already aware of the circumstances because of their membership of the Disciplinary and Penal Cases Committee would now participate in judgment of the same case – a procedure seen to be unsatisfactory over the years. Eventually (though not until the Nurses Act of 1969) the law ensured that, if a case were to go right through the professional disciplinary system, it would be subjected to the consideration of two entirely separate groups of members.

The records of the Disciplinary and Penal Cases Committee over the early years of the life of the former General Nursing Council for England and Wales make fascinating reading, as do the Council minutes which record the charges against those referred for possible removal of their names from the register and the decisions that resulted from those hearings. They present a fragment of rather specialised social history, and reveal something of the attitudes of the members of this new registered profession to their allegedly delinquent peers.

As in the previous edition of this book, I draw attention to the first 30 cases considered by the Committee, most of which were referred on to the Council for hearing. You must derive your own conclusions as to whether the judgments made were harsh or lenient, whether they were those required for public protection or rather to pronounce a moral judgment or to punish the nurse.

Theft from shops

We tend to assume that 'shoplifting' is a phenomenon of post-Second World War society and the emergence of tempting displays in large department stores and supermarkets. It might seem surprising, therefore, that 12 of the first 30 cases (in the 1920s) involved theft from shops. Five resulted from the theft of hats from the same large London store. The remainder involved yet more ladies' hats and other items of clothing.

Eleven of the 12 respondent nurses were removed from the register. The remaining one – a deputy matron – received powerful mitigating support from the matron, the chairman of the hospital board (a magistrate) and senior medical staff. Such evidence of rallying to the aid of a convicted nurse rather than dismissing her instantly was rare in those early days of nurse registration.

Cases concerning personal conduct

Seven of the first 30 cases mentioned above were concerned with the personal conduct, completely separate from their places of employment, of the persons about whom the complaints were made. Four of the seven were removed from the register. Their 'offences' were, respectively, 'bearing two illegitimate children', 'living in adultery', 'misconduct with a man in an hotel', and 'drunk and disorderly in a public place'. Two of the remaining three were formally warned about their behaviour. One had been reported for 'betting in a public house' and the other for 'making an unauthorised collection for a good cause'. The remaining nurse had no action taken against him following a report that he had left his wife. The reader might care to compare the cases in this list with the information provided in Appendix 1.

Cases concerning patients or their property

Three cases only fell into this category. All culminated in removal from the register. One involved the theft of a diamond ring and £5 (a large sum of money in 1925) from a patient. The others involved theft of money from the property of deceased patients.

Cases concerned with employment

One nurse was removed from the register for forging a character reference to support her application for a nursing post. The other two respondent nurses in this category were also removed from the register, one for being drunk on duty and the other for being found asleep on night duty.

Cases involving theft from employers or colleagues

Three further nurses found their names removed from the register for offences of this kind. One concerned theft from her employer (of food that she argued would otherwise have gone to waste). The other two were the result of theft from colleagues – a dress and a watch respectively.

Other cases

The remaining two nurses to feature in the first 30 cases to be considered by the former General Nursing Council for England and Wales were also the subject of 'removal from the register' decisions. The first was the result of the theft of £11 from some family friends. The second, and the last of the 30 cases to which I am referring in this short retrospective study, was the first to involve drugs in any way. The particular offence is described in the Council's records as 'taking and unlawfully possessing morphine'.

A number of conclusions can be drawn from reference to the first 30 cases. Two that leap from the page are that the removal rate was high (86%) and that many of those removed were so 'removed' for reasons which had little or nothing to do with their professional work.

On the latter point, I noted with great interest that, as early as case 3 (the first reported hat theft) the Council was subjected to pressure from one of the major nursing membership organisations of the day. Its secretary wrote that the Council *must* remove this lady from the register '. . . to maintain the purity of the profession. . .'. She was removed, and the phrase 'to maintain the purity of the profession' slipped into the Council's language when notifying removal and remained there for many years to come.

I found it surprising, as I researched this subject, that certain of the types of case that were culminating in removal from the register in the period up to 1930 were still being similarly resolved in the 1940s. For example, one nurse was removed from the register in 1943 in that '. . . being unmarried, she gave birth to a child'.

The fact is, however, that a regulatory system had been established and brought into operation. It might be felt that I am implying criticism of those charged in the early years of nurse registration with determining whether a person should lose or retain the right to practise. My response to that would be to say that I imagine that those involved as Council members probably had opinions that were not unlike those of society at large. It seems clear that the context in which an incident occurred was not generally taken into account in those early years. This steadily changed during ensuing years, thus enabling the Council's members and senior professional officers to exert considerable influence on the form of the relevant clauses of the Bill that became the Nurses, Midwives and Health Visitors Act 1979.

The exertion of such influence extended not only to seeking legislation that improved the means by which the profession could regulate itself in the public interest. It was also aimed at replacing the silence and ambiguity of the old legislation with a mandatory requirement to establish and improve standards of professional conduct and the power to give advice to that end. That pressure succeeded. The importance and impact of the change has given to the system and procedures of professional regulation a new and positive emphasis.

REFERENCES

[1] *Nursing and Midwifery since 1900.* Edited by Allan and Jolley. London: Faber and Faber. Particularly Chapter 2 by R.H. Pyne; Chapter 14 by E.A. Bent.

[2] *History of the General Nursing Council for England and Wales, 1919–1969* (1969). By E.R.D. Bendall & E. Raybould. London: H.K. Lewis and Co.

[3] *A History of the Nursing Profession* (1960). By B. Abel-Smith. London: Heineman Educational Books Ltd.

[4] *The Work of Mrs Bedford Fenwick and the Rise of Professional Nursing* (1973). London: The Royal College of Nursing.

Chapter 4

New Statutory Structures, New Systems, New Opportunities

In April 1979 the Nurses, Midwives and Health Visitors Act 1979[1] received the Royal Assent and thus became law. As with many other Acts of Parliament, it did not come into operation immediately. The new statutory bodies which that law required were established by Ministerial order in shadow form during 1981. The purpose of this was to enable them to assess the requirements and opportunities of the new legislation, develop proposals for subordinate legislation on which to consult with the professions, undertake that consultation and generally prepare for a transition from old organisations to new which would be as free of disruption and as immediately positive as possible. Meanwhile the statutory and other training bodies which were to be replaced, since the various sections of the law by which they were established had effectively been repealed, pending determination of a handover date, were required to continue to fulfil their statutory responsibilities in respect of training, examinations, registration and professional discipline.

HANDOVER

The date for the new statutory bodies to come fully into operation, bearing the responsibilities and performing the functions prescribed by the Nurses, Midwives and Health Visitors Act 1979, was eventually determined by Ministerial order to be 1 July 1983. Therefore the repeal of the legislation which had established the General Nursing Council for England and Wales, the General Nursing Council for Scotland, the Northern Ireland Council for Nurses and Midwives, the Central Midwives Board for England and Wales, the Central Midwives Board for Scotland and the Council for the Education and Training of Health Visitors became effective at midnight on 30 June 1983. At the same time the Ministerial orders which, some years earlier, had established the Joint Board for Clinical Nursing Studies (for England and Wales) and the Committee of Clinical Nursing Studies (for Scotland), both responsible for post-registration courses, were withdrawn.

THE NURSES, MIDWIVES AND HEALTH VISITORS ACT 1979

This Act of Parliament introduced a new structure. The introductory paragraph to the Act describes it as:

'An Act to establish a Central Council for Nursing, Midwifery and Health Visiting, and National Boards for the four parts of the United Kingdom; to make new provision with respect to education, training, regulation and discipline of nurses, midwives and health visitors and the maintenance of a single professional register; to amend an Act relating to the Central Council for Education and Training in Social Work; and for purposes connected with those matters.'

The Act, then, required the establishment of a new Central Council. This new council took the title of the 'United Kingdom Central Council for Nursing, Midwifery and Health Visiting', thus declaring at once that its concern was with the whole of the United Kingdom and the three professions named.

The functions of the new Council are described as follows in Section 2 of the Nurses, Midwives and Health Visitors Act 1979:

'(1) The principal functions of the Central Council shall be to establish and improve standards of training and professional conduct for nurses, midwives and health visitors.

(2) The Council shall ensure that the standards of training they establish are such as to meet any Community obligation of the United Kingdom.

(3) The Council shall by means of rules determine the conditions of a person's being admitted to training, and the kind and standard of training to be undertaken, with a view to registration.

(4) The rules may also make provision with respect to the kind and standard of further training available to persons who are already registered.

(5) The powers of the Council shall include that of providing, in such manner as it thinks fit, advice for nurses, midwives and health visitors on standards of professional conduct.

(6) In the discharge of its functions the Council shall have a proper regard for the interests of all groups within the professions, including those with minority representation.'[2]

Further functions concerning important aspects of professional regulation are to be found in subsequent sections. These deal with such important matters as the means by which persons can achieve registration as a nurse, midwife or health visitor,[3] the maintenance and use of the professional register,[4] and removal from the register.[5] It can be readily seen from this list of functions in Section 2 of the Act and the major issues covered by the other sections referred to that this is legislation that is concerned with public protection and the wider public interest. It is not intended to protect the professions, or enhance their status, though both of these things might be beneficial by-products of its correct operation.

The Act also required the° establishment of a National Board for Nursing, Midwifery and Health Visiting for each of the four countries of the United Kingdom. The functions of the boards are succinctly described in Section 6 as follows:

'(1) The National Boards shall in England, Wales, Scotland and Northern Ireland respectively—

(a) provide, or arrange for others to provide, at institutions approved by the Board—

(i) courses of training with a view to enabling persons to qualify for registration as nurses, midwives or health visitors or for the recording of additional qualifications in the register; and

(ii) courses of further training for those already registered;
(b) ensure that such courses meet the requirements of the Central Council as to their content and standard;
(c) hold or arrange for others to hold, such examinations as are necessary to enable persons to satisfy requirements for registration or to obtain additional qualifications;
(d) collaborate with the Council in the promotion of improved training methods; and
(e) carry out investigations of cases of alleged misconduct, with a view to proceedings before the Central Council or a committee of the Council for a person to be removed from the register.
(2) The National Boards shall discharge their functions subject to and in accordance with any applicable rules of the Council and shall have proper regard for the interests of all groups within the professions, including those with minority representation.'[6]

MEMBERSHIP OF COUNCIL AND BOARDS

While approving legislation to establish the new Council and National Boards, Parliament also laid down the basic requirements concerning the membership of those bodies. The resulting membership structure is somewhat complex.

In each country of the United Kingdom there is a National Board. The membership varies from a minimum of 35 members (Northern Ireland) to a maximum of 45 members (England). Two-thirds of the members of each board (i.e. 24–30) are elected for a 5-year term. The remaining members (i.e. 11–15) are appointed by relevant government ministers to satisfy Section 5(5)(6) of the Act. This states that the appointed persons shall be:

'made from among persons who either (1) are nurses, midwives, health visitors or registered medical practitioners or (2) have such qualifications and experience in education or other fields as, in his opinion, will be of value to the Board in the performance of its functions.'

Even were all the appointed members to be persons who were not nurses, midwives and health visitors, practitioners from the professions would constitute a majority. In practice some of the appointed member places have been used by the Secretary of State, after relevant consultation, to appoint further practitioners to achieve a balanced membership.

Each of the National Boards then nominates seven of its members to concurrent membership of the Central Council. To that membership of 28 there is then added a further 17 members who are appointed by the relevant government minister (the Secretary of State for Health), again after appropriate consultation.

It would appear that the intention was to create a corporate structure in which the determination of educational policy and its effective implementation was rendered relatively simple, since 28 of those responsible for determining such policy are members of the Boards which are responsible for its implementation. The seven members from each Board, however, are a small minority of the Board membership. That can sometimes create difficulty and tension for those with dual membership. The greater problem that such members experience, however, is the practical difficulty of trying to find sufficient time to contribute fully to the work of both Council and Board while, at the same time, holding full-time salaried posts.

CONTINUING RESPONSIBILITIES

It can be seen from the sections of the Act in respect of professional education and training, whether for the purposes of achieving registration or thereafter, that the Council is responsible for the determination of the policy, while the Boards are responsible for carrying that policy into effect.

It can also be seen that, in respect of the investigation and consideration of allegations of misconduct, the Boards have been given responsibility for performing a sieving function, while the Council is responsible for the conduct of hearings and the decisions to remove from certain practitioners their right to practise in their chosen profession.

NEW CHALLENGES – NEW OPPORTUNITIES

The most innovative aspect of the Nurses, Midwives and Health Visitors Act 1979 was that it set down in legislation a new, challenging, forward looking, standards-related tone and the requirement that the prescribed functions be performed against this more positive backdrop. There can be few sentences in British law to compare with Section 2(1) of the Nurses, Midwives and Health Visitors Act 1979, to which I again draw attention:

> 'The principal functions of the Central Council shall be to establish and improve standards of training and professional conduct for nurses, midwives and health visitors.'

In a sentence of only 25 words, set out on the face of an Act of Parliament, our legislators have used those important words *principal, shall* and *improve*. There can be no doubt that this is legislation that is not about going backwards or simply standing still. It is most certainly about going forward.

It is not the purpose of this book to elaborate upon the work undertaken by the Council to satisfy the requirements of the Act concerning preparation for registration or for the maintenance of competence beyond registration. The Council's case for change and specific proposals concerning the former can be found in *Project 2000 – A New Preparation for Practice*.[7] Proposals in respect of competence are set out in *The Report of the Post-Registration Education and Practice Project*.[8] It is emphasised, however, that standards of preparation cannot be divorced from subsequent standards of conduct. Members of Parliament have done the professions (with which the Nurses, Midwives and Health Visitors Act 1979, is concerned) a service by placing *training* and *conduct* together in a phrase, thus reminding them that the training is not an end in itself but preparation for a very important role.

While elaboration of the requirements concerning *training* will not be found in this book, such elaboration concerning *conduct* certainly will. The next chapter concentrates on the ways in which the opportunity and challenge provided by the Act has met a response. Suffice it for the present to state that, 12 years after it was passed into law, the professions have yet to grasp fully the significance of this existing and positive Section 2(1).

REFERENCES

[1] *Nurses, Midwives and Health Visitors Act 1979*. London: HMSO.
[2] Ibid: Section 2.
[3] Ibid: Section 11.
[4] Ibid: Section 10.
[5] Ibid: Section 12.
[6] Ibid: Section 6.
[7] *Project 2000 – A New Preparation for Practice* (1986). London: UKCC.
[8] *Report of the Post-Registration and Practice Project* (1990). London: UKCC.

Chapter 5

Accentuating the Positive

The challenge and opportunities provided by the Nurses, Midwives and Health Visitors Act 1979, were being responded to even before the appointed day of 1 July 1983 when the new Central Council was to replace the previous registration and regulatory bodies.

The members of the professions had not previously been consulted by their registration bodies. Having overcome the surprise they felt at actually being asked for their opinions about a range of important matters relevant to their professional practice, they responded in steadily increasing numbers and with enthusiasm to a sequence of consultation documents. It was apparent that new channels of communication were opened through which information and opinions flowed both from and to the Council and that by this a new spirit of co-operation was developed.

An improved climate of this kind was clearly going to be essential if the Council was to fulfil that mandatory requirement placed upon it by Section 2(1) of the Act that, as one of its principal functions, it was required to establish and improve standards of professional conduct. At least this new Council, unlike its predecessors, was helped by a clause in the Act that left it in no doubt of its authority when it came to the giving of advice to persons on its register. Section 2(5) of the Nurses, Midwives and Health Visitors Act 1979, states:

'The powers of the Council shall include that of providing, in such manner as it thinks fit, advice for nurses, midwives and health visitors on standards of professional conduct.'[1]

So not only was the outcome that had to be achieved – the establishment and improvement of standards of professional conduct – clear, but the law now contained specific reference concerning one of the means by which that outcome was to be achieved.

CODE OF PROFESSIONAL CONDUCT

Thus it was that, in readiness for day one of its real life (1 July 1983), the Council prepared the first edition of an important new document. That first edition was entitled the *Code of Professional Conduct for Nurses, Midwives and Health Visitors*. A copy was enclosed with the registration documents of each person being admitted to the Council's register from 1 July 1983 onwards. Bulk supplies were dispatched to managers of nurses, midwives and health visitors and to senior educationalists with the request that they be distributed to registered practitioners. In very little time this succinct little document in a bright red cover

25

became the subject of articles and letters in the professional journals and numerous meetings to explore its implications for practice.

One of the first to go into print in the journals was Annie Altschul. In her article 'Shout at the Minister' she wrote:

'The effect on patients of nurses who feel harassed and who know that no matter how hard they work, they are unable to give proper standards of care, is rarely documented and used as evidence to those who are in positions of power.

The duty to do this is now quite openly laid on every nurse by the United Kingdom Central Council for Nursing, Midwifery and Health Visiting. Every nurse now has in her possession the Code of Professional Conduct.

The duty of every trained nurse is absolutely clear. She is accountable for her own action and responsible for the work of her subordinates. If she carries on in spite of being short staffed or inappropriately staffed, without letting those higher in the nursing hierarchy know, she is personally accountable and patients and the public in general should be encouraged to demand that she is held accountable.'[2]

In issuing that edition of its Code of Professional Conduct the Council indicated that it intended to review the contents annually and produce a revised text if it was deemed necessary. The Council also stated, in a brief notice to all registered nurses, midwives and health visitors that followed the text of the Code, that it expected members of the profession to recognise it as their responsibility, as well as the Council's, to reappraise the relevance of the Code to the professional and social context in which they practise. Further to that, it was stated that the Council would welcome suggestions and comments for consideration in its periodic review.

Bearing in mind the fact that, until only a few months before July 1983, practitioners of nursing, midwifery and health visiting had not been in the habit of having their opinions sought by their registration body, the response was astonishing. Over 4000 practitioners bothered to put pen to paper. In excess of 4000 letters were received, each providing the view of a number of practitioners (from as few as two to in excess of 30) who had discussed the text together. All of that was in addition to the expected and welcome comments submitted by the major professional organisations and trade unions with nurses, midwives and health visitors in membership. With only very rare exceptions, the comments were favourable and the suggestions constructive.

When a small group of members and professional officers of the Council assembled to undertake the promised review of the Code of Professional Conduct in September 1984 the material on which to base their discussions was composed not only of their own views and those expressed by the Council, but the constructive criticisms and suggestions of several thousand practitioners. The first edition of the Code may have been the Council's, but the professions were so involved in the contribution of the material that was considered in the first review that ownership of the second edition had, to a substantial degree, transferred to the members of those professions.

The result of the review was the publication, in November 1984, of the second edition of this important document, now deliberately entitled the *Code of Professional Conduct for the Nurse, Midwife and Health Visitor*. Although subjected to further periodic review, the second edition remains the definitive text. It reads as follows:

Each registered nurse, midwife and health visitor shall act, at all times, in such a manner as to justify public trust and confidence, to uphold and enhance the good standing and reputation of the profession, to serve the interests of society, and above all to safeguard the interests of individual patients and clients.

Each registered nurse, midwife and health visitor is accountable for his or her practice, and, in the exercise of professional accountability shall:

1 Act always in such a way as to promote and safeguard the well being and interests of patients/clients.

2 Ensure that no action or omission on his/her part or within his/her sphere of influence is detrimental to the condition or safety of patients/clients.

3 Take every reasonable opportunity to maintain and improve professional knowledge and competence.

4 Acknowledge any limitations of competence and refuse in such cases to accept delegated functions without first having received instruction in regard to those functions and having been assessed as competent.

5 Work in a collaborative and co-operative manner with other health care professionals and recognise and respect their particular contributions within the health care team.

6 Take account of the customs, values and spiritual beliefs of patients/clients.

7 Make known to an appropriate person or authority any conscientious objection which may be relevant to professional practice.

8 Avoid any abuse of the privileged relationship which exists with patients/clients and of the privileged access allowed to their property, residence or workplace.

9 Respect confidential information obtained in the course of professional practice and refrain from disclosing such information without the consent of the patient/client, or a person entitled to act on his/her behalf, except where disclosure is required by law or by the order of a court or is necessary in the public interest.

10 Have regard to the environment of care and its physical, psychological and social effects on patients/clients, and also to the adequacy of resources, and make known to appropriate persons or authorities any circumstances which could place patients/clients in jeopardy or which militate against safe standards of practice.

11 Have regard to the workload of and the pressures on professional colleagues and subordinates and take appropriate action if these are seen to be such as to constitute abuse of the individual practitioner and/or to jeopardise safe standards of practice.

12 In the context of the individual's own knowledge, experience, and sphere of authority, assist peers and subordinates to develop professional competence in accordance with their needs.

13 Refuse to accept any gift, favour or hospitality which might be interpreted as seeking to exert undue influence to obtain preferential consideration.

14 Avoid the use of professional qualifications in the promotion of commercial products in order not to compromise the independence of professional judgement on which patients/clients rely.

The change in the title of the document from the plural to singular, no longer addressing the profession globally but each person on the Council's register individually, was deliberate and is deserving of explanation. Within weeks of the distribution of the first copies of the first edition it began to become clear that numerous practitioners seemed to have decided that it applied to other people but not to them. In particular it seemed that some nurses, midwives and health visitors in management positions believed that it applied only to those in more junior posts than themselves. Recognition that this attitude problem existed led not only to the change in the title but to the use of the word 'Each' to open both the introductory paragraph and also the stem sentence from which the subsequent 14 clauses grow.

The second edition – the *Code of Professional Conduct for the Nurse, Midwife and Health Visitor* – has stimulated many people within the profession, either individually or with others, to engage in an exploration of its implications for their practice and the settings within which they practise. They have been assisted in this endeavour by the fact that the Code, either directly or through issues growing out of it, has been the subject of numerous conference papers by this author and other people, has provided the basis of many professional seminars, has received attention through a number of published articles (e.g. references 4 and 5) and is the subject of an excellent book.[6]

The UKCC, having been required by the law that established it to establish and improve standards of professional conduct and to give advice on such standards, produced the Code in response to that requirement. That, however, is only part of the story. The Code was also produced for three other specific reasons:

(1) To establish more clearly than ever before the extent of the accountability of registered practitioners.
(2) To assist practitioners in the exercise of their professional accountability so as to achieve high standards of professional practice.
(3) To encourage practitioners to assert themselves so that the primacy of the interest of their patients and clients is respected.

For these additional reasons it is important to note that the Code opens with an unequivocal statement. There can surely be no doubt after reading the introductory paragraph that the primacy of the interests of the patient and client provides the first theme of the Code and establishes the point immediately that, in determining his or her approach to professional practice, the individual practitioner should recognise that the interests of public and patient must predominate over those of practitioner and profession. To assert this repeatedly and, of course, to act it out in various ways is to recognise that, for the nursing, midwifery and health visiting professions, power comes most from promoting the interests of those it exists to serve.

The Code is, then, a statement which draws attention to and emphasises the primacy of the interests of the patient or client. It has also, not unreasonably, been described as something of a statement of the profession's values. What else can be said of it? For the purposes of this book, three other definitions are offered. First, that the Code is a portrait of the practitioner the Council wishes to see within the profession. Second, that it constitutes, for nurses, midwives and health visitors, something of an extended definition of 'accountability'. Thirdly, that it now provides the backcloth against which allegations of misconduct made against practitioners and which call into question their registration status are judged.

The Code as a portrait

If you look at the Code as a portrait, what sort of portrait do you see? I hope that you find, as I do, that the introductory paragraph provides the answer to this question. It is saying, is it not, that this is the portrait of someone who acts so as to justify public trust and confidence, to uphold and enhance the good standing and reputation of the profession, to serve the interests of society, and to safeguard the interests of patients and clients. The words of that introductory paragraph describe no sinecure. Having, however, been of value in their own right, they have continuing value in that they provide the framework for the remainder of the document. Once again I wonder, when you look at the Code as a portrait, what sort of portrait do you see?

Surely one which supports my contention about the primacy of the patient's/client's interests, since it is there either overtly or implicitly in every one of the clauses. Surely this is a portrait of a person who is a professional in his or her own right, both equipped and willing to recognise the direct responsibility that goes with such a status. Surely this is a portrait of a person whose concern for patients means that they will not silently tolerate the intolerable and that they will be articulate in their representations about those things which obstruct the delivery of good care, place patients or clients at risk, jeopardise standards or endanger colleagues.

The Code not only focuses attention on the patient or client, but provides a set of sound principles on which professional practice can be based so as to ensure that his or her interests can be properly served.

The Code as an extended definition of 'accountability'

The message to registered nurses, midwives and health visitors is that this important document is really all about being accountable – all about professional accountability and its implications. It may seem surprising, therefore, that the words 'accountable' and 'accountability' each occur only once in the text. The significant point is where they are located. They are to be found in the stem sentence out of which all the subsequent clauses grow. They thus provide the central focus of a document which is built upon the expectation that practitioners will conduct themselves in the manner it describes and will do so because it is manifestly in the interests of those they serve.

Although there are some practitioners who may seek to convince the reader, as others like them have sought to convince this author, that 'accountability' is some kind of optional extra, it is clearly an integral part of professional practice. In the course of his or her professional practice, each practitioner has to make judgments in a wide variety of circumstances and has to be answerable – able to be called to account – for those judgments. The Code of Professional Conduct seeks to assist practitioners by setting down an important set of principles.

This key document does not, therefore, seek to say everything that there is to be said in fine detail. One of the important things that it does state, however, is that all practitioners who are on the Council's register are expected to seek to set and achieve high standards and thereby to honour the requirements of its first clause.

There are those who seek to denigrate the status and importance of the Code of Professional Conduct by emphasising that it is not part of the law. In that particular sense they are correct. What matters, however, is the background of law out of which it has grown. That background requires the Council, as one of its mandatory functions to establish and improve standards of professional conduct. It also empowers the Council to give advice to practitioners, in such manner as it thinks fit, on standards of professional conduct. The situation in law is therefore quite clear. The Code of Professional Conduct stands on firm legal ground.

The stem sentence in the Code out of which all the subsequent clauses grow is worded:

'Each registered nurse, midwife and health visitor is accountable for his or her practice and, in the exercise of professional accountability, shall:'

That short sentence, completed in turn by each of the numbered clauses (which should never be cited detached from their stem) is of great significance as advice to practitioners. It is significant first because it says to each practitioner that *You* (because it says each nurse, midwife and health visitor) are accountable for your practice. It states that, in the exercise of professional accountability, you shall do the things set out in the 14 clauses that follow, because that is necessary in the interests of patients or clients, directly mentioned in seven of the clauses and the obvious reason why the other seven are there. It is also significant for its emphasis that *You* are accountable for your practice – not someone else acting as your proxy. The link to clause 2, for example, is very important. You are accountable for what you do, for what you fail to do and for what happens within your sphere of influence.

The emphasis placed upon the latter definition cannot be overstated. There are still too many practitioners who have not grasped the size and nature of their personal professional accountability. There are still too many practitioners who are unaware of their own vulnerability. There are still too many practitioners who allow themselves to be lulled into slack practices which cast good standards aside and create risks for patients. There are still too many practitioners who accept delegated functions without sufficient information in the distorted belief that the delegator continues to bear the responsibility. These points apply irrespective of the practice setting and as much to the professional manager or teacher as to those in direct clinical practice. They are not made to encourage negative or defensive practice, but to emphasise the point that it is only by being a true professional in your own right, living up to your profession's standards of personal accountability and drawing attention to those things which carry risks to patients/clients and cast good standards aside that you can create an environment that is really good for patients and clients. (Some of the case studies in Chapters 12 and 13 illustrate the dilemmas associated with the exercise of accountability and the consequence of failure in this respect.)

The Code as the 'misconduct' backcloth

One further way of describing the Code is that it is now the backcloth against which allegations of misconduct in a professional sense are judged. It seems entirely reasonable that, having given advice to practitioners on its register as to what it expects of them in matters of conduct, the Council should measure alleged misdemeanours against the background of exactly that advice. Within weeks of its publication the Code quickly became a substantial feature of Professional Conduct Committee hearings when the committee members had to decide whether they regarded any facts that had been proved, when considered in their particular context, to constitute misconduct in a professional sense. If it is reasonable for that committee to use the Code as a yardstick in that way, it is simply a matter of enlightened self-interest for practitioners to use it to assess the acceptability of their own conduct.

Further advice

The Code of Professional Conduct, while continuing to be the central feature, is certainly not the Council's only advice to its practitioners on what is expected of them. Advice is provided in response to the very large number of people who write, telephone or call at the Council's offices. Advice is provided through the many study days, seminars and conferences at which the Council's professional staff present papers or contribute to workshops and discussion groups. Advice is provided in documents distributed by the Council to people on its register.

Confidentiality

As a response to perceived need the Council published, in 1987, a special advisory document to elaborate upon clause 9 of the Code of Professional Conduct. This advisory paper 'Confidentiality: An elaboration of Clause 9 of Second Edition of the UKCC's Code of Professional Conduct for the Nurse, Midwife and Health Visitor'[1] is reproduced as Appendix 3.

Exercising accountability

The set of advisory documents was further extended in 1989 when the document entitled 'Exercising Accountability'[7] was published. This document (which is reproduced as Appendix 2) explores the link between the Code of Professional Conduct and the subject of accountability. It then goes on to consider a number of important 'accountability' issues, including 'Concern in respect of the environment of care', 'Consent and truth', 'Advocacy on behalf of patients and clients', 'Collaboration and cooperation in care' and 'Objection to participation in treatment'. It concludes by listing a set of principles against which to exercise accountability. The last of these emphasises that the practitioner should be able to justify any action, or decision not to act, taken in the course of professional practice.

Other specific documents

The advisory documents referred to above have been supplemented by a number of papers dealing with specific issues. They include widely distributed statements on 'AIDS and HIV Infection' and 'Advertising and Commercial Sponsorship'.

From all of this, and the 'Aspects of Accountability' studies in Chapter 13, it can be seen that the liberating aspects of the Nurses, Midwives and Health Visitors Act 1979 have been used and continue to be used to positive advantage. There was a strong tendency in the past for 'good conduct' to be identified as being compliant and submissive. That unfortunately still holds good for many in the nursing, midwifery and health visiting professions. The practice is changing, however, as more practitioners reject that view and realise instead that 'good conduct' involves being honest, open, questioning and challenging, because those qualitites – linked, of course, with knowledge, skill and compassion – are those that best serve the interests of patients and clients.

It remains necessary, of course, to keep in place a system and procedures for considering the continued right to practise of the few within the profession who become the subject of allegations of misconduct. Fortunately, in parallel with that system, there now exists, in accordance with the law, a requirement that standards of professional conduct will be established and improved and an overt power to give advice to help achieve such improvement. The emphasis really is on the positive.

REFERENCES

1 *Nurses, Midwives and Health Visitors Act 1979*, Section 2(5). London: HMSO.
2 Altschul A. (1983) Shout at the Minister. *Nursing Mirror* 5 October 1983.
3 *Code of Professional Conduct for the Nurse, Midwife and Health Visitor.* (1984) London: UKCC.
4 Pyne R. (1986) Tell me honestly. *Nursing Times* 21 May 1986.
5 Pyne R. (1988) On being accountable. *Health Visitor* **61**.
6 Burnard P. & Chapman C. (1988) *Professional and Ethical Issues in Nursing.* London: John Wiley.

Chapter 6

Investigating and Judging Alleged Misconduct

The introductory paragraph of the Nurses, Midwives and Health Visitors Act 1979, describes that piece of primary legislation as:

'An Act to establish a Central Council for Nursing, Midwifery and Health Visiting, and National Boards for the four parts of the United Kingdom; to make new provision with respect to the education, training, regulation and discipline of nurses, midwives and health visitors and the maintenance of a single professional register; to amend an Act relating to the Central Council for Education and Training in Social Work; and for purposes connected with those matters.'

Section 12 of the same Act of Parliament states:

'1. The Central Council shall by rules determine circumstances in which, and the means by which:

   (a) a person may, for misconduct or otherwise, be removed from the register or part of it, whether or not for a specified period;
   (b) a person who has been removed from the register or a part of it may be restored to it; and
   (c) an entry in the register may be removed, altered or restored.

2. Committees of the Council shall be constituted by the rules to hear and determine proceedings for a person's removal from, or restoration to, the register or for the removal, alteration or restoration of any entry.

3. The Committees shall be constituted from members of the Council; and the rules shall so provide that the members of a committee constituted to adjudicate upon the conduct of any person are selected with due regard to the professional field in which that person works.

4. The rules shall make provision as to the procedure to be followed, and the rules of evidence to be observed, in such proceedings, whether before the Council itself or before any committee so constituted, and for the proceedings to be in public except in such cases (if any) as the rules may specify.

5. Schedule 3 to this Act has effect with respect to the conduct of proceedings to which this section applies.'

It is within the general framework of that introductory paragraph and in fulfilment of the specific requirements of Section 12 that the United Kingdom Central Council for Nursing, Midwifery and Health Visiting (UKCC or the

Council) prepared the subordinate legislation, the current editions of which are found in Statutory Instrument 1987 No. 2156 (for England, Wales and Scotland) and Statutory Instrument 1987 No. 473 (for Northern Ireland). This subordinate legislation (known as 'The Professional Conduct Rules'), before becoming law, required the approval of the Lord Chancellor (for England and Wales), the Lord Advocate (for Scotland) and the Lord Chief Justice in Northern Ireland.

These statutory rules establish, with considerable precision, not only how the requirements of Section 12 of the Nurses, Midwives and Health Visitors Act 1979, are to be satisfied, but also those of Section 6(1)(e) of the same Act. The latter clause concerns the investigation of allegations of misconduct said to be of 'professional' concern.

The Act established not only the UKCC but, in each country of the United Kingdom, a further statutory body called the National Board for Nursing, Midwifery and Health Visiting. The function of the Boards is primarily that of taking, within the framework of UKCC policy, the necessary executive action concerned with the education and training of nurses, midwives and health visitors. The Act, at Section 6(1)(e), however, also placed with the National Boards the responsibility of investigating allegations of misconduct and deciding whether the practitioner whose alleged misdeeds had been the subject of such investigation should be referred for hearing to the UKCC's Professional Conduct Committee.

In March 1989, management consultants commissioned by the Government Health Departments to conduct a review of the UKCC and National Boards established by the Act after 5 years of operation, submitted their report to Ministers. In that report they recommended a number of significant changes. One of the most significant is that the investigation of allegations, like the judgment of those requiring hearing, should rest with the UKCC and not with the National Boards. At the time of completion of this manuscript the Government's response to the management consultants' report is still awaited. The change referred to, like several other recommendations, would require amendment of the Nurses, Midwives and Health Visitors Act 1979, and therefore that rare commodity – Parliamentary time. Should the recommendation be accepted and new legislation be approved and brought into effect, although the statutory body responsible for the work will change, the method is unlikely to vary significantly.

I therefore focus attention on the committees responsible for the sieving and judgmental stages respectively (the Investigating Committee and Professional Conduct Committee) rather than on the National Boards and the Council. The reader who requires a fuller explanation of the roles, functions and sources of membership of those statutory bodies can find that I have provided a detailed description elsewhere.[2] Suffice it for the purposes of this chapter to state that nurses, midwives and health visitors form a significant part of the membership of both Boards and Council. The important principle of the profession regulating itself in the public interest is therefore honoured.

COMPLAINTS ALLEGING MISCONDUCT

The law is written in such a way that it is open to any person to bring to the attention of the Council an allegation that a person on its register has, through something he or she had done or has failed to do, raised questions about their appropriateness to retain that registration status and consequent right to practise. The Council has published (in 1990) a document to assist potential complainants understand both the system for dealing with allegations of misconduct and those which suggest unfitness to practise due to illness. This document ('. . . with a view to removal from the register . . . ?') is reproduced as Appendix 1.

INVESTIGATION

The publication mentioned above contains (in its Annexe A) a flow diagram which explains, in simplified form, the process by which an allegation of misconduct is considered. From the diagram it can be noted that the complaints which require investigation and subsequent consideration come from two sources.

Findings of guilt in criminal courts

One source of complaint is the criminal courts. Systems exist in each of the four countries of the United Kingdom which seek to ensure that, where a person known or believed to be a registered nurse, midwife or health visitor has been found guilty of a type of offence that may raise questions about his or her future registration status, a formal notification is submitted so that the matter may be given due consideration.

The notification of a finding of guilt having been received, it is then necessary to obtain from the officers of the relevant court a certificate of conviction or a certificate of the adjudication of the court. The effect of Section 13 of the Powers of the Criminal Courts Act 1973 is that a 'true conviction' is only deemed to exist if the court, having established guilt through either the defendant's admission or by hearing convincing evidence, then imposes an actual penalty. These take the form of an actual or suspended prison sentence, a monetary fine, a community service order or (in Scotland only) an admonition. If the person, having been found guilty, is then made the subject of an absolute or conditional discharge or a probation order no penalty is deemed to have been imposed by the judicial system. While a notification of the finding of guilt should be submitted where the offence is of a relevant kind, further proceedings cannot be taken by other bodies based on that finding alone. It is necessary to assemble evidence of witnesses to be called should the case be referred for Professional Conduct Committee hearing and the person not admit to the charge or charges.

In those cases where the criminal court hearing has concluded with a 'true conviction' the assembly of evidence is relatively simple. A certificate of conviction from an appropriate officer of the court which heard the case is proof of the facts of which the person was convicted and he or she is not allowed to go behind that conviction. This fact emphasises how essential it is that registered professional practitioners (in any profession) should not plead guilty in court if they are not, since that plea may have profound effects on their professional career.

This illustrates how one section of the law can affect the operation of another. Faced with two nurses who have pleaded guilty to exactly the same offence and who have similar mitigation to offer, one group of magistrates may fine the nurse appearing before them a small sum of money (therefore a true conviction) while another may make their guilty nurse the subject of a probation order. The statutory bodies can deal with both cases, though the second only at greater cost and inconvenience. Provided guilt has been established it is the offence and not the penalty that determines whether the case should be reported.

In addition to obtaining a formal certificate of conviction, it is usual, in investigating a conviction case, to obtain a statement from a relevant police officer as to the circumstances leading up to the conviction.

The very existence of the reporting system referred to above reinforces the status of nursing, midwifery and health visiting in the United Kingdom. The general (and I believe totally reasonable) philosophy behind this practice is that policemen, magistrates or even judges cannot properly determine what is of concern to a particular profession, but rather that such matters should be considered and determined largely by members of that profession sitting in collective professional judgment.

OTHER ALLEGATIONS

The second source of reports concerns people on the UKCC's register who have not appeared in court and been found guilty, but whose conduct is perceived by others to be so unsatisfactory as to question seriously their appropriateness to practise, believing vulnerable members of society to be unsafe in their hands.

The majority of such allegations concern incidents occurring in the course of professional practice. They may be by professional or general managers who have already taken a decision to dismiss a practitioner from his or her employment, but who, after consideration, take the view that the conduct that led to that decision also raises serious questions about that person's appropriateness to practise with patients or clients at all. They may be made by professional colleagues (often quite junior and recently qualified colleagues), sometimes only after their own managers have responded in what they regard as an inadequate way to serious complaints taken to them in the interest of patients and supported by clear evidence. They may be brought to the attention of the regulatory body by patients, their relatives or other visitors, or by any individual who feels concerned about something he or she has observed.

It is, then, any person's right to complain about any nurse, midwife or health visitor. Whether that person is a professional manager, a colleague, a patient or someone else, that right in this matter is still the same. It is incumbent on the statutory body, having received a complaint, to investigate it with the same zeal and thoroughness, irrespective of the source.

It must, of course, be the case that no practitioner can have his or her name removed from the register and thus be prevented from practising on the basis of another person's unproven statements and allegations. Those allegations must be thoroughly investigated and tested, no matter what the cost in time or money. It is to assist people in this potential complainant category particularly that the UKCC has published and distributed the document found at Appendix 1.

The formal complaint alleging misconduct is but the beginning of the process. It is then necessary to have the complaint investigated. This will involve identifying those people who were present at the time and place of an alleged incident and can be called to give evidence should the case be referred for professional conduct hearing. This stage of assembly of the evidence is very important. Statements must be obtained from those who will be or may be called in evidence, it being recognised that the standard of evidence is that of the criminal courts and not the much lesser standard (giving credence to hearsay evidence, etc.) of employment disciplinary proceedings.

THE PRACTITIONER'S STATEMENT

It is essential of course, to obtain both sides of any story. Therefore, as well as assembling all the available evidence in support of allegations against a practitioner, the written response of that practitioner to the allegations is sought. The process is the same where there has been a conviction. These documents together form the material which will be considered by the Investigating Committee.

THE INVESTIGATING COMMITTEE ROLE

As the flow diagram in Annexe A of Appendix 1 indicates, the Investigating Committee has three options from which to choose. A number of the statutory body's members who have accepted the onerous responsibility of serving on the Investigating Committee will have considered the papers individually in advance. They now assemble to convert their individual reactions to the information before them into a collective professional judgment.

Unlike their predecessors with the former statutory bodies prior to July 1983, if they see evidence that the conduct that has resulted in an allegation of misconduct may be indicative or symptomatic of illness, they can decide to direct the case into a more appropriate channel, where the health of the practitioner can be considered. (That system is the subject of Chapter 7.) If the view is taken that the problem is one of conduct rather than illness, two choices remain.

If the members believe either that there is insufficient evidence to prove the allegations against a named practitioner, or that (even if proved) the facts are not such as to warrant removal of the practitioner's name from the professional register, a decision to close the case will be made and no further action will be taken in respect of those allegations. If, on the other hand, the members believe that there is evidence to substantiate the allegations and that, if proved, removal from the register must be regarded as a distinct possibility, the case will be referred for a hearing before the Professional Conduct Committee. The practitioner will be advised, in writing, after the Investigating Committee consideration of the case, which of the three decisions has been made.

THE NOTICE OF INQUIRY

There can be very few letters received by any practitioner which match in significance that which formally notifies him or her of the hearing which might culminate in removal from the register. The statutory rules prescribe the wording of the letter into which the specific charges and information as to time and place are inserted. This states:

'Take notice that the charge(s) against you, particulars of which are set forth below, has(have) been brought to the notice of the Council, and that the Professional Conduct Committee of the Council proposes to investigate such charge(s) at a meeting to be held at . . . and to determine whether your name should be removed from the register or any part or parts of it.

You are hereby required to attend before the Professional Conduct Committee of the Council at the time and place mentioned above and to answer such charge(s), bringing with you all papers and documents in your possession relevant to the matter and any persons whose evidence you wish to lay before the Professional Conduct Committee.

It should be carefully noted:

You are entitled to be represented at the hearing before the Professional Conduct Committee by a friend (including a spouse or other relative), or by counsel or a solicitor, or by any officer of a professional organisation or trades union, but if you propose to be so represented, you should give written notice to the Registrar of the Council at the address mentioned above at least seven days before the Hearing.

A copy of the Nurses, Midwives and Health Visitors (Professional Conduct) Rules 1987 is enclosed.'

Before that letter is sent the practitioner who is to become the respondent in the case (and their chosen representative if formal notification has been given that there is one) will have received other communications. First, he or she will have received a letter advising that the case has been referred for a hearing. Second, if it is a case other than a true conviction, copies of the statements of the witnesses who are to be called to give evidence are sent so that the respondent is made fully aware of the case he or she has to defend. Third, the respondent is sent a copy of the evidence which has been assembled about his or her previous history and which it is intended be called and submitted only if both the facts alleged and misconduct are proved to the required standard.

THE PROFESSIONAL CONDUCT COMMITTEE HEARING

Since the whole purpose of professional regulation is that the interests of the public must be protected from unsafe practitioners, this must be particularly the case with hearings before the Professional Conduct Committee.

It is in recognition of this fact that the committee meets in public. This makes it possible for members of the public to attend, observe and form a view as to whether the profession is regulating itself in such a manner as to serve the public interest. Access of this kind is facilitated by the committee meeting not only at its London headquarters but also in venues around the United Kingdom dependent on the geographical distribution of cases.

Although the principal purpose of the public hearing is that stated above it serves an important secondary purpose. Many members of the profession choose to attend as observers. With few exceptions they report it as being a salutary learning experience which sends them back to their own workplace with their eyes newly opened to some of the hazards they had previously accepted without question.

The Professional Conduct Committee convened for the hearing of a case is made up of five members of the Council, selected (as the law requires) with due regard to the practitioner's professional field.

THE STAGES OF THE HEARING

There are four specific and separate stages of a hearing which follow the formal reading of the charges and a plea in response. The first is concerned with establishing whether that which is alleged to have happened can be proved. The second is to determine whether any facts which have been established constitute misconduct in a professional sense. The third is to receive evidence about the previous history of the respondent and for him or her to offer evidence in mitigation. The flow diagram indicates the sequence of events but cannot contain explanations of a number of important points.

In the third 'Did it happen?' stage, the standard of evidence is that applying in criminal courts. That is to say that only direct evidence is regarded as admissible and hearsay or second hand evidence is not. It also means that it is not permitted for either a representative or the Council's solicitor to ask the witnesses leading questions, i.e. questions which imply the answer. This may sometimes result in an allegation that was found proved in a disciplinary hearing of a health authority not being proved before the committee. A legal assessor (a barrister, advocate or solicitor of at least 10 years standing) sits with the committee to ensure that the rules concerning admissibility of evidence and other matters of law are observed, but does not participate in the decision making.

Just as the standard of evidence is strict, so also is the standard of proof. It is not sufficient that the committee members think that the matters alleged probably happened. In order to find the facts alleged in any charge proved the members must be satisfied to the degree of being sure. Mere probability will not suffice. No lesser standard would be acceptable when the committee has in its power a sanction as enormous as that of removing a person's right to practise in his or her chosen profession.

If the facts alleged in one or more charges against a respondent are proved to the required standard the committee must then decide whether those facts are to be regarded as misconduct in a professional sense. Before doing so the respondent or representative is given further opportunity to address the committee and to call further evidence. The Council's solicitor is unlikely to call further evidence, recognising that the case is being heard by a committee that has the relevant expertise within its membership. In deciding whether the facts are to be regarded as misconduct in a professional sense, the committee will consider those facts in the context of their occurrence rather than in isolation. The members will also have regard to the advice given by the Council regarding expected standards of conduct (in its Code of Professional Conduct) and to the definition of misconduct in the Professional Conduct Rules. The latter states that 'Misconduct is conduct unworthy of a nurse, midwife or health visitor.'

If misconduct is proved in respect of any of the charges, the committee must then receive information concerning the respondent's previous history. The Council's solicitor, through evidence or other assembled material, will provide factual information concerning any previous criminal convictions, findings of misconduct or formal disciplinary action.

The respondent can then submit any evidence in mitigation he or she has assembled. This may take the form of further witnesses called to testify as to the respondent's character or written documents.

Only when all of that is completed will the committee retire, to consider in private which of the judgments available to it is appropriate to the case.

PASSING JUDGMENT

As with the Investigating Committee, the Professional Conduct Committee, if it takes the view that the matters before it are or may be a product of illness, can transfer the case into the other channel which will consider medical evidence (see Chapter 7). If that course of action is not taken there are three options from which the members of the Professional Conduct Committee can choose.

Postponement of judgment

Ultimately the respondent practitioner's name must either be removed from the register or not be removed. The law provides a third but essentially interim solution which is to postpone its judgment on the misconduct the committee has had proved to its satisfaction

If the committee decides to postpone its judgment it means that the respondent's name remains on the register and that he or she can apply for or hold any post for which the relevant qualifications are held. It also means, however, that the person must appear again before a committee which still has the option of removal from the register to use if it deems it necessary in the public interest. Therefore, in announcing a decision to postpone judgment in a case, the committee chairman must also indicate the period of postponement and any criteria that the members wish to see satisfied during that period.

At a resumed hearing the committee, again meeting in public, is presented with information concerning the facts that were established and found to be misconduct in a professional sense. References from persons nominated by the respondent are also received. The law requires that the persons nominated as referees must be aware of the facts previously established and must have known the respondent practitioner during the period of postponement. Reports (e.g. from the Nurses' Welfare Service, probation officers, etc.) are also received. On the basis of all of this information the committee members then question the practitioner before allowing him or her a final opportunity to address them in further mitigation. The committee then retires to arrive at its decision.

Removal from the professional register

At either a first hearing or a hearing resumed at the end of a period of postponed judgment, the Professional Conduct Committee has the same three options from which to choose. If postponement of judgment is discarded the committee, meeting in private, next considers whether to remove the respondent's name from the Council's register. If it so decides the decision is immediately effective. A decision to remove a practitioner's name from the register is never taken lightly. It is an enormous sanction. The person has been admitted to the room as a registered nurse, midwife or health visitor, or possessed of registration in more than one such category, and now leaves the room no longer possessed of that status. The making of such a decision is an uncomfortable burden to bear, but the members recognise that, at the point of making it, they act on behalf of the entire registered profession and with the interests of the vulnerable public to the fore.

Misconduct proved but no further action

If the committee rejects the postponed judgment option and decides that the proved misconduct, when considered in context and in the light of the respondent's previous history and general character, does not necessitate removal from the register, the case is closed. That should not be regarded as an indication that the committee condones or regards as acceptable the actions or omissions it has both proved and regarded as misconduct. Nor should it be interpreted as an indication that the respondent has been, in any way, 'let off'. He or she, in a public hearing, has been found guilty of misconduct in a professional sense by a committee of his or her peers. That finding will be held on record for 10 years and will be brought forward as important antecedent history if, at any time within that period, the practitioner is found guilty of further misconduct.

ANNOUNCEMENT OF THE COMMITTEE'S JUDGMENT

The wording of the statutory rule governing the announcement of the committee's decision requires that the chairman announce the decision in whatever terms the committee determines. This passage of subordinate law is extremely important, since it means not only that (whatever decision has been made) a public comment can be made about the respondent practitioner's conduct, but comment can also be passed concerning the setting in which the incident(s) occurred, where that is appropriate. This can often serve to make an apparently surprising decision not to remove a person's name completely understandable.

APPEAL AGAINST REMOVAL

Given the enormity of the ultimate sanction available to the Professional Conduct Committee it is neither surprising or unreasonable that Section 13 of the Nurses, Midwives and Health Visitors Act 1979 allows that 'A person aggrieved by a decision to remove him from the register . . . may, within 3 months after the date on which notice of the decision is given to him by the Council, appeal to the appropriate court. . .'.

The UKCC, like the statutory regulatory bodies for other professions, has found its decisions challenged in the courts more frequently than was the experience of the former statutory bodies. It should not be assumed from that statement that it is a common occurrence, but nine cases in 6 years is a high rate compared with the two appeals against the decisions of the former General Nursing Council (for England and Wales) Disciplinary Committee in its 64 years of existence. The increase in the number of appeals would appear to be a product in part of the greatly increased number of cases being heard, but it is clear that it is also an indication that society at large adopts a more challenging attitude to bodies on which Parliament has conferred substantial powers.

JUDICIAL REVIEW

It is not only through appeals tabled under the terms of Section 13 of the Act that the courts have become involved in examining specific cases heard by the UKCC's Professional Conduct Committee. Judicial review is a growing area of law and has been used by a small number of practitioners to obtain a review by a judge or judges of a hearing in which, though not removed from the register, the matters alleged against them were proved and regarded as misconduct.

In a minority of the relatively small number of appeal or judicial review cases, those bringing the case have succeeded in having the finding against them set aside. Whatever the outcome, a critical reading of the verbatim transcript of the case by the judges, supplemented by the kind of question and answer process that is a feature of such hearings, has aided a review and some revision of both the committee procedures and statutory rules. For example, different legal assessors took a different view of what might be regarded as admissible under the requirement on the Council's solicitor to present '. . . evidence as to the previous history of the respondent.' Two appeal cases in which it was alleged that prejudicial material was admitted at that stage served to clarify the matter. This does not necessarily occur, since on some other matters the view presented by the judges in one case has been significantly different from that presented on the same issue by other judges in a second case. It is clear, however, that the judges are reluctant to interfere with the decision of a professional committee charged with the onerous burden of considering cases brought against members of their profession without good reason.

RESTORATION

Removal from the register is not necessarily the end of a person's career as a registered nurse, midwife or health visitor. Indeed, for some it appears to mark the beginning of a necessary professional rehabilitation, the need for which was only recognised when the removal decision was announced.

Section 12(1)(c) of the Nurses, Midwives and Health Visitors Act 1979 provides the basis in primary law for restoration to the register as well as removal from the register.

A person whose name has been removed from the register may make application for restoration as and when he or she so decides. Arrangements then have to be made to hear and consider the application before the Professional Conduct Committee. Before that can take place, references in support of the application must be obtained from persons nominated for that purpose by the applicant. The procedure at the hearing is similar to that described for hearings resumed at the end of a period of postponed judgment. The committee must simply either accept or reject the application.

THE WORKLOAD

The Professional Conduct Committee work makes very large demands upon the members of the Council. In the six-year period from April 1984 to March 1990 inclusive the committee sat on 558 days. In the course of those hearings, 954 new cases, 122 cases resumed at the conclusion of periods of postponed judgment and 208 applications for restoration were considered.

Of the cases that were concluded during that same period 399 persons were removed from the register, 89 were placed on postponed judgment, 369 had misconduct proved but were not removed, 17 were referred to the Health Committee, 151 applications for restoration were accepted and 57 similar applications were rejected.

In that same period the Committee sat, in public, in venues ranging from Inverness in the North to Plymouth in the South and to Harlech in the West. A genuine effort has been made both to enable members of the public to see how these professions respond to the requirement to regulate themselves and members of the profession to derive positive lessons from this ostensibly negative activity.

REFERENCES

1 *Nurses, Midwives and Health Visitors Act 1979.* London: HMSO.
2 Pyne, R.H. (1984) Managing the Profession. In *Managing Nursing,* edited by R. Rowden. London: Baillière Tindall.

Chapter 7

Unfitness to Practise due to Illness

INTRODUCTION

In the early paragraphs of the previous chapter the words of Section 12 of the Nurses, Midwives and Health Visitors Act 1979 were drawn to the attention of the reader. It is that passage of the primary law that allows subordinate law ('rules') to be made concerning the circumstances in which and means by which a person may be removed from the professional register.

There is one significant respect in which this passage in present law differs from the comparable passage in the law that established the former statutory bodies (for nursing and midwifery) and governed their proceedings. The old and now repealed laws referred only to establishing rules whereby '. . . a person may, for misconduct, be removed from the register.' The British Parliament, in its wisdom, replaced this with a passage which refers instead to removal from the register '. . . for misconduct or otherwise. . . .'

The change was welcomed by those previously involved in operating the law concerning the regulation of nursing and midwifery. All too often they had found themselves in possession of reports about practitioners who were clearly dangerous but about whom they could do nothing since those practitioners, though manifestly unsafe, had done nothing culpable which might be construed as 'misconduct'. All too often, sometimes after incidents with serious or even tragic consequences, they had found themselves using the awesome power of the statutory body's disciplinary machine and a public hearing to deal with someone whose basic problem was their illness.

It had been noted that the 1978 Medical Act had conferred on the General Medical Council not simply a power to consider cases in which it was believed that the fitness to practise of a medical practitioner was seriously impaired by illness but a requirement that it establish and operate the necessary committees and procedures. It was laid out in considerable detail in the primary legislation.

The General Nursing Council for England and Wales, being the statutory body then existing for much the largest number of registered practitioners of nursing, midwifery and health visiting, and consequently having the biggest Disciplinary Committee caseload, pressed for similar powers, but indicated its preference for a clause in the forthcoming Bill which would simply be enabling in nature and provide for maximum flexibility in subsequent rule making.

That request for flexibility was satisfied beyond expectations by the simple inclusion of the words '. . . or otherwise . . .' after 'misconduct' in the clause concerning removal from the register. Those two new words were to prove quite sufficient as a hook in primary legislation on to which the new Council could hang a new set of rules and procedures. It would, as hoped, be possible to enhance the protection afforded the public by allowing the Council to consider reports suggesting that certain practitioners were unfit to practise due to illness.

SAMPLING THE PROFESSION'S OPINION

It was clear, therefore, that the largest of the statutory bodies soon to be replaced had formed the view that a system to protect the public from the practitioner who was unsafe due to illness was necessary. What did the new body (the UKCC) think? Would it choose to use the flexibility provided for it by the Nurses, Midwives and Health Visitors Act 1979?

During the shadow period in which the old and the new bodies overlapped (the old continuing to run things while the new prepared for the future) the UKCC, through one of its working groups convened to examine specific aspects of the new Act, decided that the opportunity provided for it should be grasped. It put this matter as a suggestion to members of the profession through a widely circulated consultation document and found that it received wide support. As a result, the subordinate legislation was prepared and an entirely new aspect of professional regulation came into operation in 1984.

As with the procedures for dealing with allegations of misconduct, those for considering alleged unfitness due to illness are explained in the document '. . . with a view to removal from the register?'[1] which is reproduced as Appendix 1. Annexe B of that appendix provides a flow diagram to illustrate, in simplified form, the process by which such complaints or expressions of concern are considered.

REFERRAL FROM INVESTIGATING COMMITTEE OR PROFESSIONAL CONDUCT COMMITTEE

It has already been explained that if, at any stage of their proceedings, the Investigating Committee or Professional Conduct Committee form the view that the practitioner whose case they are considering is one whose fitness to practise is seriously impaired by illness, they may transfer the case in order that this view be tested through medical examinations and subsequent consideration by the Health Committee.

THE PANEL OF PROFESSIONAL SCREENERS

As the flow diagram indicates, such referred cases, once the necessary documentation has been assembled, are referred to a group of UKCC members known as the Panel of Professional Screeners. This panel is composed of 12 members, only three of whom are normally assembled to consider any set of cases.

In cases referred by either of the committees in the professional conduct channel, since these members have decided that the person should proceed to medical examination and then consideration by the Health Committee, the only role of the screeners is to select the categories of examiners to whom he or she should then be referred.

Once the screeners have made their decision, the practitioner who is the subject of a case is advised that the referral has been made and invited to undergo medical examination by two of the Council's specifically appointed examiners and at the Council's expense. There is no compulsion on the practitioner to accept that invition, but if he or she refuses it needs to be recognised that the Health Committee members before whom a hearing will be conducted may infer something from that refusal.

Experience since these procedures came into operation has shown that a majority of practitioners referred by either of the committees in the professional conduct channel accept the invitation and attend for medical examinations.

MEDICAL EXAMINERS

The medical examiners who serve the Council and the public interest are appointed in accordance with arrangements established by a Schedule of the Professional Conduct Rules. This section of legislation prescribes and lists the medical organisations authorised to nominate specialist registered medical examiners with a view to appointment by the Council. These, in summary, are the various medical Royal Colleges and certain committees of the British Medical Association.

When the nurse, midwife or health visitor referred to the Health Committee in the way described accepts the invitation to medical examinations, arrangements are then made for him or her to be seen by appropriate types of specialists as determined by the screeners. They will be examiners who are remote from both the practitioner's domestic or work settings to ensure an objective approach. To assist them, however, reports will be obtained in advance from the person's general practitioner and any specialist by whom he or she has previously been treated, provided that consent is given for this to be done.

THE PRACTITIONER'S OPTION

The medical examiners submit very detailed medical reports to the relevant UKCC staff. Copies of the reports are then sent to the practitioner about whom they have been written so that he or she is fully aware of the contents of what will be the key documents before the Health Committee. It is then open to the practitioner to decide whether, either with the support of a professional organisation, trades union or other professional adviser, or as a personal decision, to commission one or more further reports from specialists of their own choosing. Sufficient time is allowed both for consideration of this matter and for any further medical examinations to be concluded and the resulting reports prepared and submitted.

As a result of this activity it becomes possible, well in advance of an actual Health Committee hearing, to prepare and circulate a comprehensive document. In the case of a person referred from the Investigating Committee or Professional Conduct Committee, in addition to all the medical reports assembled, any relevant material that was before the referring committee will be included since this may provide some evidence of what might be called symptomatic behaviour.

Since the actual Health Committee hearing is conducted in accordance with the same legally determined procedures irrespective of the source of the referral, I will defer any explanation of it until I have first provided information about the other category of cases – those known as 'direct referral' cases. I do so because there are some significant differences in the procedures that precede the Health Committee hearing.

DIRECT REFERRAL CASES

Just as any person has the right to allege that a person on the Council's register is guilty of misconduct in a professional sense and have that thoroughly investigated and competently judged, so also may any person express concern that a practitioner's fitness to practise is seriously impaired by illness and to the danger of his or her patients or clients. These are known as direct referral cases.

Such cases begin with a letter from a concerned individual to the UKCC. That individual will often be a fellow nurse, midwife or health visitor in a management position, but may equally well be a colleague or a private individual. A case of this kind is only formally opened when that original expression of concern is given formal legal status in the form of a statutory declaration. The Council's solicitor therefore takes the original communication and any documents which accompanied it, prepares the statutory declaration and conveys it to the originator to sign if its contents are agreed. The purpose of this procedure is to ensure that the person initiating the case is mindful of the serious nature of the proceedings and the fact that the outcome might be the removal of the practitioner indicated from the professional register.

The screeners in direct referral cases

The role of the panel of screeners is larger in direct referral cases. At a first consideration of the available material (i.e. the statutory declaration and any annexed documents) the members assembled will first have to consider whether there is any evidence of illness of a significant nature. If they take the view that there is not they can close the case immediately and require that both the originator of the case and the practitioner be so advised. If they believe there to be cause for concern that has to be pursued they select the category (or categories) of medical examiners to be used.

The arrangements for such examinations are the same as in the first category of cases. What is different, however, is the power that is invested in the screeners in direct referral cases. Whereas in cases referred by one or other of the committees in the professional conduct channel the panel of screeners' role is limited to selecting the categories of medical examiners, it is not so here. The screeners are asked to consider the case again with the benefit of the reports prepared and provided by the Council's medical examiners and any additional medical reports. Possessed of what is a substantial amount of medical evidence (in those cases in which the practitioner agreed to be examined), the members of the panel of screeners must then decide either that there is no evidence to indicate that the practitioner's fitness to practise is seriously impaired or that there is such evidence. If the former applies they close the case and notify those involved accordingly. If the latter applies the case is referred for hearing before the Health Committee of the Council.

THE HEALTH COMMITTEE

As is the case with proceedings before the Professional Conduct Committee, those applying for the Health Committee are set out in detail in Statutory Instruments 1987 No. 2156 (for England, Wales and Scotland) and 1987 No. 473 (for Northern Ireland). There are a number of significant differences which it is important to note before considering how the committee is composed and operates.

The pool of members from which, under current law, any particular Health Committee is convened is made up of 25 members of the Council. From these members a committee of five is assembled, the quorum below which the number cannot fall being three members. As with the Professional Conduct Committee, every attempt is made to pay due regard to the practitioner's field of work in assembling a committee.

Hearings in private

Unlike the Professional Conduct Committee, the Health Committee meets in private. The ultimate function of both committees is the protection of the public. It is argued by some that, this being the case, the public should have equal access to both hearings in order to be satisfied about the manner in which the Council exercises its regulatory authority. While being mindful of that argument, the Council, in exercising its rule-making authority, decided that hearings should be in private since the evidence to be received was not that of alleged culpable behaviour but the fine detail of a person's medical history and reports on their current condition. The view was taken that to have public meetings of the Health Committee would inevitably result in breach of confidentiality and would run counter to the rehabilitative influence the Committee might often exert on those appearing before it.

The fact that the meetings are held in private renders the role of the legal assessor even more important. His or her role is to advise the committee on the admissibility of evidence and matters of law in circumstances in which no public or press comment on the conduct of the case can ever be possible.

The medical examiner role

The statutory rules that govern the Health Committee proceedings require that at least one of the Council's medical examiners who has examined the practitioner and prepared a report must attend to answer questions from that practitioner (or representative) and the Committee and to act as a medical adviser in respect of other information or evidence that emerges in the course of a hearing. If the practitioner so requires, both of the Council examiners involved will attend. Where the practitioner has declined the invitation to undergo medical examinations by Council examiners, one of those who would have been used attends the hearing in the role of medical adviser.

Preparing for the hearing

It is regarded as a matter of great importance that, well before the hearing, the practitioner is sent copies of the entire set of documents that will be before the Committee, when it hears that person's case. This enables him or her, either personally or by taking advice from a professional organisation, trade union, friend or legal adviser, to decide whether to allow the hearing to proceed on the basis of the documentary evidence and medical reports or to require the attendance of relevant people to give oral evidence. With only a small number of exceptions the practitioners, recognising that the medical reports are the most important documents in the set, decide that they do not require the attendance of witnesses. Those who do are often the subject of direct referral cases and have not agreed to be examined by Council examiners.

The hearing

In those cases where oral evidence is required the proceedings are broadly similar to those of the Professional Conduct Committee. That is to say that each witness is questioned first by the person calling him or her (i.e. the Council's solicitor or the practitioner/representative), is then cross-examined and finally questioned by the committee. The difference lies in the fact that what the committee must determine, having heard evidence of the symptomatic behaviour giving rise to the complaint, is whether the practitioner's fitness to practise is seriously impaired by illness or not.

In the other cases (where oral evidence is not required) the hearing is based around the assembled documents. In cases referred by one of the committees in the professional conduct channel these will include, in addition to the medical reports, the documents which were before that committee. In direct referral cases the statutory declaration recording the expression of opinion that a practitioner may be unfit to practise, together with any appended witness statements, is included.

Every attempt is made to keep hearings of this kind as informal as is possible and consistent with the fact that, at its conclusion, those who make up the Committee may announce a decision to remove the practitioner's name from the register.

After introductions have been effected the Committee's chairman formally draws attention to what the statutory rules call 'The grounds for belief that the practitioner's fitness to practise may be seriously impaired by a physical or mental condition'. That done, the attending medical examiner draws attention to points of particular significance in the medical reports and then responds to questions about those reports from the practitioner (or representative) and the Committee.

The practitioner is then questioned by the Committee members. If the practitioner is assisted by the attendance of his or her own medical adviser, that person is then able to address the Committee and answer the members' questions. The attending medical examiner, now cast in the role of medical adviser, is then requested to advise the Committee about any points of significance identified in the course of the proceedings. Finally the practitioner or representative addresses the committee before it retires to make its decision.

Committee decision

The Committee must choose from a range of four decisions. At one extreme it can decide that the practitioner's fitness to practise is seriously impaired by illness. If it so decides it must remove the practitioner's name from the register. No matter how sympathetic the members may feel towards the practitioner, this is the action the law requires be taken in the public interest.

At the other extreme the Committee can decide that the practitioner's fitness to practise is not seriously impaired by illness. The use of the present tense in the previous sentence is significant. It may well emerge that the practitioner's fitness was seriously impaired at some time in the past and that such impairment led to the actions which became the subject either of allegations of misconduct to the Investigating Committee or direct referral. If the Health Committee decides that the practitioner's fitness to practise is not (definitely) seriously impaired by illness it must close the case. In a small number of cases referred by either the

Investigating Committee or the Professional Conduct Committee it emerges that no evidence of illness at the time of the actions or omissions that resulted in allegations of misconduct and which might explain them can be found. In these cases the Health Committee will refer the case back to the Committee whence it came for the 'misconduct' issue to continue to be addressed. It cannot refer to either of those committees a case which began as a direct referral.

Between those extremes the Committee can either postpone its judgment for a stated period or adjourn the hearing for further medical reports. When it takes the former course of action it must indicate the medical evidence it will require for the resumed hearing. When it takes the latter decision it is often because the available medical evidence is contradictory, ambivalent or ambiguous. In such a case the hearing can be resumed as soon as the further medical evidence becomes available. At the resumed hearing of either type of case the procedures are similar to those at the original hearing.

Right of appeal and application for restoration

The right to appeal to the relevant court which has been explained in Chapter 6 also applies to the person aggrieved by a 'removal' decision of the Health Committee. So also does the right to apply for restoration to the register. In the latter case the Health Committee hearing the restoration application will require the medical reports specified by the Committee which ordered removal. If satisfied from the medical evidence that the person is again fit to practise he or she will be restored to the register.

THE SYSTEM IS JUSTIFIED

The architects of the Panel of Professional Screeners and Health Committee system have good reason to be pleased with what has been achieved. The protection afforded to the public has undoubtedly been enhanced. In addition to that, a sensitive system now exists which has had a profound rehabilitative effect on the lives of a substantial number of practitioners and will surely continue to do so in respect of other practitioners in the future.

The Nurses, Midwives and Health Visitors Act of 1979 established the United Kingdom Central Council for Nursing, Midwifery and Health Visiting and opened the door for it to introduce this important extension to the regulatory system. Since the Council chose to pass through that door, make the required statutory rules and bring into operation the procedures described above there has been a marked consistency about the types of cases received and considered. A majority of cases each year have been persons with alcohol-related illness. Next come other forms of drug dependence and various manifestations of psychiatric illness.

STATISTICAL INFORMATION

In the statistical year April 1989 to March 1990 the Panel of Screeners met on 13 occasions and considered 101 cases. There were 31 direct referral cases and in all of these the panel decided, at the first stage of consideration, to proceed with the case and select the category of medical examiners. At the second stage of consideration the panel referred 25 cases to the Health Committee. Six cases were closed on the grounds that the medical examiners' reports did not indicate serious impairment.

Twenty-eight cases were referred by the Investigating Committees of the National Boards and six cases were referred by the Professional Conduct Committee. The categories of medical examiners were selected by the Panel of Professional Screeners and these cases then proceeded to the Health Committee.

The panel also selected the category of medical examiners for applications for restoration to the register by the Health Committee. There were five such cases. The Health Committee met on 14 occasions and considered 81 cases. Fifty-eight new cases were heard and of these it was decided in 49 that the practitioners' fitness to practise was not seriously impaired and the cases were closed. The Committee postponed judgment on 13 cases. In 15 cases it found fitness to practise was seriously impaired which resulted in the removal of the practitioners' names from the Professional Register.

There were 19 cases which were resumed at the end of the period of postponed judgment and in all these the Committee decided that fitness to practise was not seriously impaired and closed the cases.

There were four applications for restoration to the Professional Register and these applications were all accepted.

The major reasons for referral to the Health Committee in this period were alcohol dependence (32 cases), depressive illness (23 cases), other mental illness (17 cases), drug dependence or abuse (8 cases) and ophthalmic disorder (1 case).

Chapter 8

The Role of The Nurses' Welfare Service

The existence of a welfare or support service linked to the disciplinary function of a statutory body, though still questioned by some practitioners, is now broadly accepted. The suggestion that such a step should be taken was viewed with considerable scepticism when it was first mooted in 1972. In spite of the reservations of many people at that time, the dream of a dedicated few became a reality later in the same year when the former General Nursing Council for England and Wales became the first regulatory body for any of the registered professions to both support the existence of a specialist agency and use its services.

The basic philosophy underlying its establishment was that nursing, as a caring profession, should be concerned about the relatively small yet still significant number of its members who find themselves involved in the disciplinary procedures of their regulatory body. Nineteen years on, that underlying philosophy still holds good. The major change to have occurred is that the potential clientele is now composed of all the nurses, midwives and health visitors on the UKCC's professional register – approximately 600000 people with current effective registration.

It would be all too easy to castigate the small number of practitioners who have become the subject of complaints alleging misconduct as the delinquents who have brought their profession into disrepute by their reprehensible actions. In some cases that is absolutely true. To make such judgment in respect of all such practitioners would, however, be to hide from the truth and be tantamount to an abdication of professional responsibility towards colleagues who have cracked under intolerable pressure or are victims of inadequate working environments allowed to exist by those who have now rejected them. The Nurses' Welfare Service's explanatory leaflet is appropriately entitled *When the coping becomes too much. . . .*[1] As a disciplinary case unfolds it so often becomes all too apparent that the practitioner concerned has been subjected to intolerable levels of stress, either at home, at work, or in both settings simultaneously. Of course there are exceptions, but the majority of nurses, midwives and health visitors are caring, conscientious people with a strong professional commitment. Such practitioners are not immune to the pressures that can sometimes culminate in atypical behaviour.

ORIGINS OF THE NURSES' WELFARE SERVICE

The decade that saw the birth of what became (and is still known as) the Nurses' Welfare Service was one which also witnessed a fundamental reappraisal of the whole concept of professional discipline on the part of the one council which helped that organisation into existence and assisted it to establish its important role. Suddenly a subject that had been kept fairly secret was being discussed at conferences, seminars and study days all over the country. This resulted in a significant increase in the level of awareness about the disciplinary aspect of the work of the General Nursing Council (for England and Wales). The Nurses Welfare Service played then, and continues to play, a vital part in the development of a more caring, positive, enlightened philosophy with regard to professional discipline. This philosophy is that rehabilitating an offending practitioner can be a recognised objective to pursue, while taking the action required to protect the public from unsafe practitioners.

Looking back to 1972, it can be seen that grafting a social work agency that offered support to an individual nurse involved in the disciplinary process on to the statutory body's established process was not an easy task. Extreme caution was necessary to ensure that the service was established on a firm legal base and that it would not interfere in any way with the due process of law by which that body had to investigate and judge complaints against named individuals. It is interesting to look back and note that, in its original terms of reference, the Nurses' Welfare Service, through its professional staff, could only become involved in a case after the Disciplinary Committee had made its decision. Over the next few years the role of the service was the subject of continuous review and evaluation. The result was that the remit of service was steadily extended.

The model on which this service is based is the statutory Probation and After-Care Service. There are many similarities between the two in that probation officers are social workers operating in a court setting and many of the clients of the Nurses' Welfare Service have already been convicted in court and are identified by their connection with the statutory body's disciplinary function. Experience in statutory probation work has therefore proved to be the most appropriate background for those who take posts as professional welfare advisers with the Nurses' Welfare Service.

The situation now with UKCC, as was the case until 1983 with the General Nursing Council for England and Wales, is that the relationship between the Council and the service is one of sensitivity, delicacy and mutual trust. Some people find it difficult to understand how a statutory body with responsibility for taking disciplinary action against an individual practitioner (in many cases removing their right to practice) can at the same time make possible the offer of a helping hand. Experience has shown that these two concepts are complementary rather than contradictory, provided you accept the basic premise that professional regulation and discipline is about the protection of the vulnerable public and not about punishment. It is also established as essential that the help and support offered must be, and must be perceived to be, separate from the body taking the disciplinary action, even though funded by that body in a majority of cases. This separation is vital from the point of view of potential clients, as it must be abundantly clear to them that they can enter into relationships of trust with the welfare advisers in the certain knowledge that none of the information shared in the course of an interview will be passed on to anyone without prior consent.

NURSES' WELFARE TRUST

To emphasise the separate nature of the service, a trust was established (as a registered charity) at the onset to bear the responsibility for administering the service and raise a substantial part of the money the operation requires. In a large number of cases the UKCC recognises the practitioners' need of support and also recognises that its decision making will be aided by the kind of background social enquiry reports that, with consent, will be made available by the welfare advisers. In such cases the UKCC formally commissions the work and therefore meets its full cost. The remainder of the income is obtained through voluntary donations and the support of some established charitable trusts. Such income is essential as it meets the costs of providing a service which, by counselling and support at an earlier stage, helps prevent many practitioners deteriorating to that point where report to the statutory body occurs. The number of practitioners who can be assisted is, however, limited by the funds available.

The existence of the trust (the Nurses' Welfare Trust; registered charity 266994) has given the service professional independence and ensured that its staff are accountable to and able to receive support and advice from the trustees, several of whom are respected practitioners from the social work profession. Separation from the statutory body is therefore seen to be important. So also is the existence of a close working relationship with the statutory body from which the service derives its credibility, much of its stature and its very reason for existence.

ROLE OF THE NURSES' WELFARE SERVICE

The work of the Nurses' Welfare Service underwent a dramatic and interesting expension in 1984 when the UKCC brought into operation its new procedures which allowed it to consider removal from the professional register not only for reasons of 'misconduct', but also where a practitioner's fitness to practise was alleged to be seriously impaired by physical or mental illness. The procedures for considering allegations of misconduct have been explained in Chapter 6 and those for considering possible unfitness to practise due to illness in Chapter 7. Both are the subject of further explanation in Appendix 1. Suffice it here to say that a large number of the practitioners whose fitness to practise is the subject of consideration both need and receive a great deal of specialist support during an extremely difficult and testing time in their lives. One such practitioner, who has been a client of the Service, happily now restored to the register, has very courageously told his story in an article in Nursing Times.[2]

The Nurses' Welfare Service is, therefore, a specialist social work agency, staffed by qualified professional social workers, which exists to provide casework help and support for any nurse, midwife or health visitor involved in, or at risk of becoming involved in, the disciplinary or fitness to practise procedures of the regulatory system in the United Kingdom. The fundamental premise on which the work is based is that of a voluntary contract between client and welfare adviser.

Potential clients of the service may come to its attention by self-referral, referral from other social workers (notably Probation Officers), or referral from concerned professional managers or colleagues. Many who fall in the first category make contact, having been made aware of the existence and role of the service through an introductory leaflet enclosed with the letter sent on behalf of Investigating Committee to invite a statement in respect of the misconduct alleged. Some others in that category will receive a similar leaflet when invited to attend for medical examinations because concern about their fitness to practise has been expressed. Provided that the individual practitioner gives written consent, the officer of the Nurses' Welfare Service involved with the case will be provided with copies of all relevant documents as they are assembled.

The role of the service is not that of appearing at the Professional Conduct Committee or Health Committee as a representative or advocate. That is the task of the officer of the professional organisation or trade union of which the practitioner is a member or of the lawyer the practitioner engages for the purpose. Such a representative is committed to obtaining the best possible outcome of the case for the client. The welfare adviser is concerned with endeavouring to help the client face up to the reality of the situation, even though that may be painful at the time. The files of the Nurses' Welfare Service would illustrate the large number of occasions on which it was necessary for its staff to get their clients to face up to the inevitability of removal from the register. Those same files would also illustrate how frequently the individual's acceptance of that fact marked the beginning of their rehabilitation.

There are those who, either for effect or because they are concerned that it might mislead, express concern that the word 'welfare', included in the service's title when it was first created in 1972, still remains there. It does so because the service is concerned with the welfare of individuals, both short-term and long-term. It provides a casework/counselling service for its clients, enabling them to identify the underlying factors which have brought them to their statutory body's attention. It assists clients to formulate realistic plans to work through the identified problems. It ensures that practitioners are accompanied and supported on what are among the most important yet most lonely days of their lives. It is still there to assist the practitioner when a committee of his or her peers has decided that the public interest requires that they should not be allowed to practise in their chosen profession. Surely all these are aspects of welfare, using that word in its broadest and most constructive sense.

THE WORK OF THE NURSES' WELFARE SERVICE

Much of the work of the welfare advisers is undertaken by visiting clients in their homes. Such visits tend to be particularly productive for both adviser and client. The latter normally feels more relaxed and able to talk more freely in the familiarity and security of his or her own home. The fact that the welfare adviser has probably travelled a long way for that home visit tends to be seen as demonstrating his caring attitude. The practitioner – often dismissed from employment and now at risk of losing his or her registration status – is helped by this single gesture to feel valued again.

The work is rarely easy. Indeed, it has become very clear from an early stage of the existence of the service that (for the welfare adviser) working with a client group composed of fellow professionals in what must still be regarded as a pioneering field of social work demands very special skills. Numerous nurses, midwives and health visitors have difficulty accepting that they need help. This may be because they lack insight into their particular problem – something commonly encountered where it is alcohol- or drug-related. It may be because accepting that you have a need of help tends to be seen by many practitioners as a sign of weakness or an admission of defeat. Added to that, for all of us in the caring professions, is the fact that to be receiving care is a reversal of roles.

One major focus of the work – now as in the formative years of the service – is that of short-term crisis intervention during the period that clients are actually going through the professional conduct or fitness to practise systems. Anxiety is at least partially allayed. The complexities of the system are explained. The myths and fantasies some practitioners still have about the powers of the Council are replaced by the facts.

In addition to such short-term work, each welfare adviser carries a nucleus of long-term cases. For the most part this is made up of practitioners whose names have been removed from the register by one of the two committees empowered to make this decision and who have chosen to maintain contact with the service for the advice and assistance it can give them as they seek to equip themselves for restoration to the register. This aspect of the work can be difficult and frustrating, but in the end often proves extremely rewarding. Convincing a client of the futility of applying for restoration within days of receiving the letter confirming removal from the register is a common experience for all the welfare advisers. By making a premature restoration application a client risks further rejection by his or her profession. For some, however, that further phase of rejection is necessary before they face up to the facts and start to rebuild their lives, either within their chosen profession or in some other area of work.

Social background reports

Reference has already been made to the preparation of social background reports to be presented to the committee considering the case of a practitioner who has voluntarily chosen to accept the assistance of the service. The purpose of preparing such a report is to enable the committee to see the matters which have brought the practitioner to their attention in the context of that individual's personal and professional life. On occasions a social background report reveals a catalogue of disasters of such magnitude that one is left wondering how the practitioner in question managed to keep going so well for so long. A report can also serve to indicate that the incident which has placed the practitioner's registration in jeopardy is the result of momentary aberration when under pressure and needs to be seen in the context of 20 years unblemished, committed, high quality professional service.

The assistance the members of the committees derive from these reports in the difficult decisions they have to make is enormous. Each report is a comprehensive, objective, honest appraisal of the client and his or her circumstances, prepared by someone who is knowledgeable about the committee's role and powers and mindful of its prime responsibility to protect the vulnerable public.

CASE HISTORIES

Two case histories are provided to illustrate the nature of the work of this important service. Further illustrative material can be found in the 1987/1989 *Report of the Nurses' Welfare Trust*.[3]

Case history 'A'

Susan, a 34-year-old registered general nurse, with an impeccable professional record, was employed as a sister in an accident and emergency unit at a small general hospital in a quiet provincial town. She had been in post for some five years and enjoyed an excellent reputation amongst her professional colleagues as a highly competent sister.

Following the break-up of her marriage, she became acutely depressed and turned to alcohol in an attempt to escape from the unhappy state in which she found herself. Her intake gradually increased to the point where it began to affect her performance at work. Colleagues noticed all was not well but turned a blind eye, making allowances for the difficult time Susan was experiencing in her personal life. Then one day she inadvertently administered the wrong medication to a patient. During the enquiry which followed, a bottle of sherry was discovered in Susan's changing room locker. Her dependency on alcohol had become so acute that she was unable to finish a shift without recourse to the sherry bottle.

She was dismissed from her post and reported to the statutory regulating body for investigation. At this point she made contact with the Nurses' Welfare Service, feeling she was a total failure, having lost her husband, her job and now being faced with the prospect of having her name removed from the professional register. She felt both ashamed and yet relieved that her problem had at last come out into the open. She had become isolated and withdrawn following the failure of her marriage and had experienced a great deal of guilt because of her drinking.

Susan was in need of a lot of support, especially as she did not belong to a staff organisation. The realisation that her professional qualification was at risk convinced her of the need to seek specialist help. She spent eight weeks in a detoxification unit followed by a lengthy course of psychotherapy as an outpatient. The Welfare Adviser remained in close contact, complementing the medical care she was receiving. He also assisted her in the preparation of a statement for consideration by the Investigating Committee which decided that she should be referred to the Health Committee of the UKCC.

With the help of the Nurses' Welfare Service, Susan's rehabilitation had begun. She decided to take out an option on a new career in case her name was removed from the register, and was accepted at her local polytechnic on a secretarial/business studies course. Having nursed a large number of people in the local community, she felt so ashamed and embarrassed at meeting them in the street that she dramatically changed her hairstyle in an attempt to lessen the risk of being recognised. She found it difficult to cope with the transition from the caring role of ward sister to the very different skills required for a secretarial course. She needed a lot of encouragement to persevere, especially at times when the old craving for alcohol returned. She joined Alcoholics Anonymous and found this fellowship enormously supportive and helpful in her attempts at maintaining sobriety.

According to the requirements of the Nurses, Midwives and Health Visitors' Professional Conduct Rules, she was examined by two independent medical practitioners who prepared reports for the Health Committee of the UKCC. The Welfare Adviser, who by then had been supporting Susan for nearly two years, also prepared a detailed report explaining what had been happening during that time. He concluded that Susan had tackled her problems with courage, determination and realism . . . she had come a long way in restoring her self-respect and pride. She had not had an alcoholic drink for two years and had acquired new skills to equip her for alternative employment although at times she had found the going very hard. Finally, it was his view that she had demonstrated, over a two-year period, that her rehabilitation was successfully accomplished.

Susan attended the Health Committee, which meets in private, accompanied by the Welfare Adviser. She felt very apprehensive but gave a good account of herself. The outcome was favourable and she has recently returned to nursing, a wiser and more mature practitioner after her traumatic experiences of recent years.

Case History 'B'

Sally (aged 38 had not only excelled academically in her RGN training, carrying off most of the prizes, but was regarded by all who had worked with her as an exceptionally conscientious, committed and professional practitioner. She seemed to have an unlimited capacity for work; as well as efficiently running a busy medical ward, she fitted in a demanding Open University course, and on several occasions had to nurse her elderly parents, with whom she lived, through a variety of illnesses. On one such occasion, Sally found herself having to ferry her mother, who was suffering from lymphosarcoma, to and from hospital, and the constant pressure was interfering with her sleep. Rather than approach the notoriously unhelpful staff doctor, she helped herself to eight barbiturate tablets from the ward. By the time this came to light, Sally had commenced midwifery training; she immediately resigned despite the wholehearted support of her managers, fearing that her name would be removed from the register. However, in view of her excellent references, and the many mitigating circumstances, she was allowed to retain her professional qualification.

Sally continued her career with hardly a break, quickly finding a staffing position at another hospital, and was very soon offered a sister's post there. She also began to pursue various management training courses. Again, work pressure was heavy, and her parents' needs and her academic work took up any spare time, on top of which her friends tended to use her, too, as a counsellor and adviser. However, an attempt to lessen the load by working in a quiet local nursing home did not prove satisfactory; she missed the challenge and variety of the hospital setting, and soon applied for a hospital post again. Shortly after this move, pressure began to build up on various fronts.

Firstly, Sally began to suffer various physical ailments, beginning with an acute lumbar disc leading to complications necessitating surgery. She also suffered recurrent mouth ulcers. Her mother, meanwhile, had developed an acute illness culminating in a laparotomy for the removal of a malignant cyst, and Sally spent a lot of time looking after her during her convalescence. Finally, the staffing situation at the hospital had become increasingly parlous, and Sally had constantly to cover for senior hospital staff, and frequently to act up.

When she again developed symptoms in her leg, Sally did not return to her medical advisers, but instead began to take Valium from the ward where she worked. This led to discrepancies in the ward drug register, which were eventually discovered by which time 50 tablets had been misappropriated, over a period of about six months. Sally had used the tablets in a 'sensible' manner, as if they had been prescribed. Her manager stressed that her high standard of work had never altered.

Sally had immediately resigned her post, and was, by the time the Professional Conduct Committee considered her case, working in an antique shop cum art gallery. The Welfare Adviser who had visited several times had helped her to see clearly how her attempt to be all things to all men was ultimately self-defeating and she understood that, in the end, nothing could justify the theft and self-prescription of drugs. Sally attended the Professional Conduct Committee and it came as no surprise to be told her name was to be removed from the register.

In the aftermath of that decision Sally is in need of, and is receiving, a lot of help from the Nurses' Welfare Service in coming to terms with the loss of her professional qualification. She is in a state of bereavement having lost her right to practise in her chosen profession which she had served with distinction for 17 years. She has to live with the stigma of being 'struck off', news of which had spread through her local community by means of a report in the press. Sally also feels an acute sense of failure, having let not only herself down, but also her family, friends and especially her own professional peer group to whom she had previously promised that she would never again abuse the trust placed in her as a nurse. When she reads about the current shortage of nurses she feels guilty that because of her own folly she is no longer allowed to practise. Although she is glad to have a job in the antique shop, she feels uncomfortable and sometimes embarrassed at meeting former patients and colleagues in her new role. Any mention of hospital makes her feel rejected, de-skilled, and useless.

Sally will need a lot of time to work through the pain and hurt which she now feels. She knows that she has the ongoing support of the Service for however long she may need it. Perhaps eventually she may feel ready to apply for the restoration of her name to the professional register.

CONCLUSION

The creation and development of the Nurses' Welfare Service has been a significant feature of the positive revolution that has been occurring in professional regulation over the last two decades. Many members of the former General Nursing Council for England and Wales and the present United Kingdom Central Council for Nursing, Midwifery and Health Visiting have said that they would find it very difficult to serve on those committees empowered to remove practitioners' names from the register if the service did not exist. They take support and comfort from the fact that, because realistic and understanding support is available on a continuing basis, their decision to require removal from the register is often the first step towards that individual's rehabilitation. The many nurses, midwives and health visitors who have received support at difficult times in their lives, have become suitably rehabilitated and have since given years of high quality service to their patients and clients, are excellent evidence of the need for and achievements of the Nurses' Welfare Service.

REFERENCES

1 *When the coping becomes too much....* Explanatory Leaflet. London: Nurses' Welfare Service.
2 Crabtree D. (1990) *To Hell and Back. Nursing Times* **86**, 42.
3 *Nurses' Welfare Service – Report of the years 1987 to 1989.* London: Nurses' Welfare Service.

Chapter 9

A View of the Profession

The function of the nursing, midwifery and health visiting professions is to ensure that advice, care and treatment of a high standard are provided for members of society. To this end there is merit in examining all the available evidence concerning practice, identifying within it those things which obstruct the achievement of the desired objectives, and seek for ways of clearing the perceived obstructions.

The UKCC Professional Conduct Committee's case law can provide some of that evidence. To a lesser degree so also can the Health Committee caseload. Increasingly the dilemmas voluntarily shared by practitioners with professional staff of the Council concerning their difficulties in exercising accountability supplement these other sources in an extremely helpful and constructive way. It seems worthwhile, therefore, to examine the evidence available from these three sources as a basis for some remedial action.

WHAT LESSONS EMERGE ABOUT MEMBERS OF THE NURSING, MIDWIFERY AND HEALTH VISITING PROFESSIONS?

The basic answer to this question can best be provided against the background of the UKCC's *Code of Professional Conduct for the Nurse, Midwife and Health Visitor*, both the text and origins of which can be found in Chapter 5. It has been stated in that chapter that the code is a portrait of the kind of practitioner that the Council believes to be needed in the profession. The lessons arise out of the still considerable failure of many practitioners to comply with that portrait.

This failure is not simply that of the small percentage of professional practitioners who find themselves appearing before the Professional Conduct Committee. It ought to be regarded as shared by those who, by their silence, pretence or inaction allowed situations to exist that contributed to putting them there. It ought also to be shared by those who have misguidedly opted for silent acquiescence when challenge, questioning and honest communication were required.

THE DEMANDS OF THE CODE

A major element of the failure can be identified by reference to the code's introductory paragraph. The paragraph refers to satisfying public trust and confidence, to upholding and enhancing the good standing and reputation of the profession and to serving the interests of society. In stating the expectation that each registered nurse, midwife and health visitor will act, at all times, in such a manner as to achieve all those things the Council has set all such people a big agenda full of major challenges. The challenges do not, however, stop at that point. The paragraph concludes with the key statement of expectation that the nurse, midwife and health visitor will act '. . . above all to safeguard the interests of individual patients and clients'.

It can be seen, therefore, that the practitioner is expected to recognise that he or she, while giving good care to individuals now, must also be something of a visionary, an ambassador and a person who seeks to influence events. It is surely evident from that paragraph that practitioners must not limit their understanding of patients or clients to those cast in that role at any one point in time but must see those words as also meaning those who will be cast in that role at any time in the future. Recognition of the fact will help the practitioner to maintain lofty vision and broad perspectives. Far too many practitioners allow their world to be far too small, neither influencing or allowing themselves to be influenced by what is happening elsewhere.

THE IMPORTANT STEM

Just as that introductory paragraph provides a focus against which to describe a broad and general aspect of current professional failure, so do the separate clauses of the code provide the basis for identifying some of the other lessons that need still to be learnt by many within the profession. I cannot emphasise too strongly that each of these numbered clauses effectively completes the sentence commenced by the stem sentence out of which they grow. I refer to that which states that:

'Each registered nurse, midwife and health visitor is accountable for his or her practice and, in the exercise of professional accountability shall. . .'

No single clause should be quoted detached from that stem if its full value is to be retained. Such detachment often seems to occur in the minds of professional practitioners who, as a result, fail to link their personal professional accountability with the requirements of the specific clauses.

The interest of patients and clients

Analysis of cases appearing before the Professional Conduct Committee often underlines the importance of clauses 1 and 2 of the code and the frequency with which the requirements contained within them are not met. There is surely nothing surprising about an expectation that practitioners will act always to promote and safeguard the well being and interest of patients and clients, or that they will ensure that no action or omission on their part is detrimental to the condition or safety of patients. Time and time again, however, there appears evidence of failure to undertake the work necessary to set standards, failure to undertake any audit or monitoring of the care delivered, failure to make and maintain satisfactory records and failure to ensure that those involved in policy making and financial control have an accurate picture of the importance of their decisions.

Concurrently with all of that failure, there appears evidence of too great a willingness to accept the *status quo*, slip quietly into the kind of rut which allows the intolerable to be tolerated and to adopt a stance which demonstrates that poor standards are both expected and accepted. Surely none of this is consistent with professional accountability.

Actions and omissions

It is significant that clause 2 of the Code of Professional Conduct refers not only to the practitioner's actions but to his or her omissions, and then goes on to relate those actions or omissions to '. . . his/her part or within his/her sphere of influence'. The nurse or midwife employed as the manager of a ward cannot limit his/her concern to what he/she does or fails to do. The same applies to the staff nurse in charge of a shift on such a ward. It is not, however, only those involved in direct clinical practice who are the subject of this clause. Like the remainder of the Code of Professional Conduct, it applies to everyone on the Council's register. That being the case, it must apply to nurses employed in management positions, whether in posts specifically requiring registration (as nurse, midwife or health visitor) or not.

Failure to recognise this 'sphere of influence' point is illustrated from the experience of the Professional Conduct Committee in two specific ways, the first of a general nature and the second relating to a specific case.

Communication

First, that of a general nature. All too often I have sat with the Professional Conduct Committee when it has been hearing allegations of misconduct against a person in direct patient/client care which take the form of failure to do something that should have been done. Quite frequently in such cases, as the evidence unfolds, it becomes more and more apparent that resources (human and physical) were quite inadequate to meet the identified needs and that the person's 'failure' was nothing more than a failure to achieve the impossible. All too often in such cases I have eventually (at the 'previous history' stage of a hearing) heard a member of the Committee say to the manager called to give profile evidence (who has been in the meeting room throughout, since his or her evidence was not related to the charges) that the particular setting had emerged as one in which it was impossible to give good care to all those needing it and to ask why it was like that. All too often the reply to the question has been that he or she (the respondent) '. . . did not tell me'.

The case for communication is made. So also is the point that management is not simply about waiting to be told, but about walking the job, ensuring that you know, ensuring that communication systems are in place and are used and making your staff feel important and valued.

Sphere of influence

The specific case which illustrates that practitioners in management positions are still able to be held accountable also has a particular relevance to the 'sphere of influence' point. Two respondents appeared before the Professional Conduct Committee to answer charges alleging misconduct in the course of their work. One was employed as a night sister in a large general hospital. The other was the chief nursing officer for a large National Health Service health authority. The complaint against the sister included inappropriate behaviour in patient areas which would damage trust and confidence, serious errors in the administration of medicines (including intravenous substances), the alteration of entries in controlled drug registers to conceal the errors that had been exposed and attempts to blame her own rather reckless and cavalier mistakes on more junior members of staff.

The complaint against the chief nursing officer was to the effect that he had ordered that the investigation of a complaint made by a number of registered nurses and being undertaken by other nurse managers on the order of the hospital's director of nursing service be stopped, had ordered that her suspension be lifted and had ordered in writing that she be returned to full duties including the administration of drugs without delay.

Faced with such inappropriate handling of their legitimate complaints the same nurses then brought those complaints to the statutory regulating body, culminating in the Professional Conduct Committee hearing. The chief nursing officer argued that, being remote from the clinical scene, his actions could not be regarded as misconduct in a professional sense. The Committee found, however, that by ordering the night sister's return to duty while the investigation of complaints was incomplete, he had placed at risk every patient in her care. This being established against a person on the Council's register, it seemed logical to regard it as misconduct in a professional sense. Like the sister, the chief nursing officer was removed from the register. He exercised his right of appeal, making a similar point, but the court rejected his application that it overturn the decision.

It can therefore be seen that both failure to intervene when appropriate and active intervention that is inappropriate remain features that tarnish good professional practice.

Competence and honesty

Analysis of the Professional Conduct Committee's work also underlines the importance of clauses 3 and 4 of the Code of Professional Conduct. It appears self-evident that practitioners should take every reasonable opportunity to maintain and improve professional knowledge and competence. In spite of this fact, however, there continue to be many within the profession who, it appears, take the view that, on the day that they first achieved registration status, they were equipped for all of the world and all of time, with never a need to read a professional book or journal, attend any kind of professional event or even engage in intelligent conversation with professional colleagues. I refer briefly in the penultimate chapter to the new demands and challenges that seem likely to be placed before such practitioners. Suffice it for the present to say that practitioners of the kind described fail to be the kind of practitioners that both their profession and the public have reason to expect.

Delegated functions

The same can be said of the central point of clause 4 of the Code. This requires that the practitioner will acknowledge any limitations of their competence and refuse to accept delegated functions which they are not equipped to perform until instructed and brought to a level of competence. It is unfortunate to have to state it, but all too many practitioners do not comply with this requirement. For some, this is a product of pride, fear or some other emotion. For others it is more a matter of ignorance or of simply being unaware. In either case there appears to be a strong tendency for those who fail in respect of this clause also to fail in respect of clause 3.

Collaboration and cooperation

Continuing to use the Code of Professional Conduct as a backdrop against which to comment on the evidence of sundry failures that exist and the lessons that remain to be learnt, I turn to its clause 5. This clause concerns the importance of working in a collaborative and cooperative manner with other health care professionals. Once again I stress the importance of reading this clause linked to the stem that forms the first part of the sentence. That stem emphasises that each individual practitioner bears a personal accountability and that it is in the exercise of that accountability that collaborative and cooperative working has to be achieved.

The whole clause must be read within the context of a respect for the primacy of the interests of the patient or client. It is not an invitation or encouragement to accept improperly delegated functions. It is not implying in any way that the nurse, midwife or health visitor should behave in a subservient manner in the presence of other professional practitioners, and particularly not when the interest of the patient or client requires from them an assertive intervention. It is making the point, however, that, in many situations, good quality care and treatment can only be provided by a good quality team to which all its component practitioners contribute fully.

In her hospital-based novel *Shroud for a Nightingale*, P.D. James has one of her characters state that 'Vanity is a surgeon's besetting sin, as submissiveness is a nurse's'.[1] I comment only on the second profession named. The evidence of failure to which I refer in respect of clause 5 of the code is that of willingness (in some cases almost determination) to be submissive at the very time that the patient needs the professional practitioner who has spent most time with her to recognise that the time has come to take up an advocacy role.

Customs, values and beliefs

Failure to appreciate the full significance of the stated expectation that practitioners will take account of the customs, values and spiritual beliefs of patients and clients also becomes evident. At its lowest level such failure manifests itself in an inability to recognise the importance of such matters to a particular patient or client. At the other extreme it involves a more disturbing attempt by the practitioner to impose his or her own beliefs and values on patients and to proselytise. In either circumstance, or at any point between these two extremes, it is unacceptable. It indicates that this is a matter on which the profession has much work to do.

Conscientious objection

The intention of the authors of the Code of Professional Conduct in including a clause requiring that practitioners made known any conscientious objection they may have which might be relevant to professional practice was that service to patients and clients should not be unreasonably disrupted.

For many years the only conscience clause permitting a professional practitioner to opt out of providing a particular service was found in the Abortion

Act 1967. More recently a similar clause has been inserted in the Human Fertilisation and Embryology Act 1990. These clauses are for the benefit of practitioners and respect their consciences. They also serve the interest of patients in ensuring that professional practitioners involved in the treatments to which these Acts of Parliament refer have no entrenched opposition to those treatments which might subliminally affect delivery of the treatment and associated care.

Unfortunately some practitioners seek to claim conscientious objection to participate in certain forms of care and treatment for which there is no justification. Such claims usually do no more than reveal the practitioner's own attitudes and prejudices towards patients with certain conditions and their own ignorance about those conditions.

One case (in 1990) before the Professional Conduct Committee involved a nurse who first unsuccessfully sought to argue her 'conscientious objection' case and then refused to care for a patient with acquired immune deficiency syndrome (AIDS). She would find no support for her stance in either the Code, in *Exercising Accountability* (see Appendix 2) or in the UKCC's published statement on *AIDS and HIV Infection*.[2] The second and third of these documents make the point very firmly that the Code does not provide a formula for being selective about the categories of patient for whom you will care or for being in any way judgmental. The nurse in the case referred to was removed from the register.

Confidentiality

The UKCC advisory document which elaborates upon clause 9 of the Code of Professional Conduct is reproduced as Appendix 3 and is commended to the reader. Certain of the case studies found in Chapters 12 and 13 illustrate some of the dilemmas faced by individual practitioners in respect of confidentiality. I simply state at this point that far too many practitioners have not yet grasped the importance of confidentiality and consequently fail to honour the expectations of the code.

The environment of care

The comments I have already made which have sought to assess how the professions are doing when measured against clauses 1 and 2 of the Code can be applied also to clauses 10 and 11.

It seems, all too often, that practitioners are determined to deceive themselves that they are delivering good care when they are not, to pretend that things are better than they really are and generally to conceal the truth and deny the reality which stands exposed before them. It would seem that there is a great fear in some people of making accurate records or communicating honest reports lest they be marked out as someone who cannot cope, is incompetent or is a trouble maker. Perhaps the greater concern felt by such practitioners is that, if they do draw attention to those matters about the environment of care or the pressure on their working colleagues, rather than be supported by their professional peers with similar problems they will be deserted by them. The last few years have been marked by a number of examples of exactly this.

Annie Altschul, in the article from which I have already quoted in Chapter 5, referred to this problem as follows:

'I am sure that most nurses have at times of staff shortage or of a sudden increase in the number of very ill patients given less than the best care. But they have pretended to themselves, to patients and to their relatives that all was well. They have perhaps even taken pride in managing against all the odds. Never would they have dreamed of appearing disloyal by disclosing to the public or to members of the government or to the press, that good nursing care was impossible under the circumstances.'

She later adds:

'The duty of every trained nurse is absolutely clear. She is accountable for her own action and responsible for the work of her subordinates. If she carries on in spite of being short staffed or inappropriately staffed, without letting those higher in the nursing hierarchy know, she is personally accountable and the public in general should be encouraged to demand that she is held accountable.'[3]

In writing what I have about the lessons that emerge about members of the professions regulated by the UKCC I recognise that I have tended to generalise from the particular. Since, however, the particular examples have been so numerous I have no doubt that the messages they bring can be generally applied and that it would be unwise to ignore them.

WHAT LESSONS EMERGE ABOUT HEALTH CARE MANAGERS AND EMPLOYING AUTHORITIES?

I have written at some length about what I have perceived to be the failures of practitioners and I have cited in aid the writings of one senior member of my profession whose views I respect. I readily accept, however, that those who manage and those who employ nurses also contribute to the situations I have described. To put what I have said in context I list a number of respects in which I believe managers and employers, on occasions, also fail, in the hope that some critical self-examination may take place as a result.

Stress and pressure

There is the responsibility which both managers and employers bear for the delivery of safe and competent care and in a manner that does not result in the staff being subjected to unreasonable pressure. It seems that, all too often, managers fail to recognise the stress to which they submit their most reliable staff. (Some illustrations of this can be found in the case studies in Chapters 12 and 13.)

Scapegoats

There is the frequently observed phenomenon, when something goes wrong, of looking for a person to cast in the role of the scapegoat to whom to attach the blame and make it appear that the entire problem has been resolved. That scapegoat is often the most junior of the qualified nursing staff. On other occasions the one person who has been a lone voice in drawing attention to the hazards of the particular setting is singled out. On rare occasions it is even the one member of staff from an ethnic minority who has erred, in common with others, but becomes the only one to be subject of significant disciplinary action.

Linked in some respect with this phenomenon is the tendency, when an individual practitioner takes action to expose a situation in which patients or clients are placed at risk or standards of care seriously jeopardised, for attention to be directed at finding fault with the individual rather than addressing the faults or problems of the institution or service.

The devaluation of direct care

Next, there is the tendency of managers to expect and indeed impose 'acting up' arrangements which often serve to pull the most experienced and knowledgeable practitioners away from the settings where care is delivered and either not to replace them or do so with an unqualified and inexperienced person. This, like numerous other occasions in which improper and inappropriate delegation is an inevitable consequence of a manager's action, or when nursing staff time is used to cover the gaps in other services, seems often to indicate that the actual delivery of care to patients and clients is regarded as of little value.

Lack of knowledge

Another matter of concern is the serious lack of knowledge sometimes manifested by professional nursing or midwifery managers whose role includes that of recruitment. A stark illustration of such lack of knowledge was manifested by the nurse managers who expected one applicant for a post in a renal unit to have a blood test for HIV because, in the ward elsewhere in which she had been working for a few months, several beds were used for the care of patients with AIDS.

The ignorance these managers demonstrated of the methods of transmission of the infection or of sero-conversion time was extremely disturbing. So also was the fact that they had not, and had no intention of expecting other staff of the renal unit to have similar blood tests. Further still, they were unaware of the difficulties that just stating you have been tested for HIV can currently cause for an individual seeking a mortgage or insurance cover.

The implications of statutory registration

There is cause for concern in the fact that some employers often seem to fail to realise that the nurse, midwife or health visitor (like any other statutorily registered health professional) cannot simply be regarded in the same way as other employees. For instance, the registered medical practitioner who engages in what the General Medical Council deems to be improper delegation may well be removed from the medical register as a result. It would therefore be unacceptable for that doctor's employer to require him to delegate any particular activity to a person who is not sufficiently knowledgeable or competent to perform it. Exactly the same principle applies to the nurse, midwife or health visitor.

In preparing and publishing its Code of Professional Conduct, the UKCC has performed a service not only for patients and the public. It has performed a service for the practitioners on its register. It has also performed a service for those who employ nurses, midwives and health visitors, since there is surely nothing in the Code of Professional Conduct which, while being the Council's expectation of people on its register, is not also a reasonable employer's expectation of a reasonable nurse, midwife or health visitor employee. The employer cannot expect a practitioner to do something or silently accept a situation which exposes him or her to the risk of complaints which question his or her continued registration status.

The ill-considered response

Yet another cause for concern is the tendency observed in some quarters, when problems have been identified, to grasp at the expedient short-term response rather than seek for a genuine long-term solution. The result of such an approach is often that short-term relief is followed by an exacerbation of the original problem.

Documentation of care and treatment

One specific area of concern relates to the subject of record keeping and the documentation of patient/client care. It has been astonishing to note that, in some situations, nurses have been encouraged or even instructed not to state goals or objectives in care plans, or to insert only very limited goals, on the grounds that recorded goals or objectives not attained can leave the health authority vulnerable to successful action for damages. One is forced to ask just whose interests are we meant to be serving?

While I recognise that the standard of records made by nurses, midwives and health visitors often leaves much to be desired and that the need for improvement is apparent, I cannot accept that practitioners should embark upon the care of a patient with severe limits imposed upon what they record about what they hope and expect to achieve from that care.

Employers and managers, like individual practitioners, need to note the significance of the Access to Health Records Act which reached the statute book in 1990 and becomes operative from November 1991.[4] From that date onwards, records concerning patient care, whether held on computer systems or in manual form, will be accessible on request to the people to whom they relate unless there is an exceptionally strong reason, in the patient's interest, to deny such access.

Standards

The final concern that I record in respect of managers and employers repeats one of those set down in respect of individual practitioners. This is the unfortunate tendency to both expect and accept poor standards.

These, then, are the concerns in respect of managers and employers that I place on record. As with that part of this chapter concerned with practitioners in general, I again recognise the unfairness that generalisations of this type can be to those who do not act in the way described. To such managers and employers I apologise.

That does not alter in any way my conviction that everyone involved – individual practitioners, managers and employers – should review their practices, procedures and policies regularly to ensure that they cannot justifiably be criticised fot the failures and in respect of the concerns described. To achieve this satisfactorily, no evidence should be ignored.

REFERENCES

[1] James P.D. (1989) *Shroud for a Nightingale*. London: Penguin.
[2] *AIDS and HIV Infection*. London: UKCC, 1989.
[3] Altschul A. (1983) Shout at the Minister. *Nursing Mirror* 5 October 1983.
[4] *Access to Health Records Act 1990* London: HMSO.

Chapter 10

The Current Law and its Operation

At the time of publication of the first edition of this book (1981) the Nurses, Midwives and Health Visitors Act 1979 had reached the statute book but had not come into operation. The effective date of operation was subsequently determined by government ministers as 1 July 1983.

In that first edition I engaged in some conjecture about the effects that this new primary legislation might have and commented upon the opportunities it offered for improvement. Before concluding this second edition I look back over seven years during which this new Act has been in operation. In doing so I comment on what I perceive to be the benefits that have resulted and also draw attention to those aspects of the Act which, in retrospect, seem to be defective, even if well intentioned.

KEY STATEMENT OF THE COUNCIL'S ROLE

On more than one occasion in the previous chapters of this book I have drawn attention to Section 2(1) of the Nurses, Midwives and Health Visitors Act and emphasised its importance. I make no apology for reiterating this point. The presence of this vitally important statement at the beginning of the section concerning the functions of the new Central Council has proved extremely beneficial. No more was there to be any doubt. The new statutory regulatory body for nursing, midwifery and health visiting was required to establish standards and also improve standards.

It can be fairly said that the Council has responded to this challenging requirement with enthusiasm, recognising fully its public service role. The first five-year membership term was marked by the publication of important documents concerned with the mandatory requirement that, as principal functions, both standards of training and professional conduct be improved.

In respect of the former the Council concluded the first phase of an enormous piece of work in May 1986 when it published the 'Project 2000' Report, *Project 2000 – A New Preparation for Practice*.[1] The Council's continued pressure to see the changes to nursing education recommended in that report become operative is steadily being rewarded as colleges of nursing undertake the preparatory work that must precede this revolution in nursing education and then admit their first students to the new style courses.

As for the latter, the Council marked its arrival on the scene with the immediate issue of its first edition of the Code of Professional Conduct and followed it up in 1984 with the second and still current edition of that important advisory document aimed at achieving improvements in standards of professional conduct. That clause (Section 2(1)) of the Act has most certainly proved worthwhile and must be protected at all costs.

ADVICE TO THE PROFESSION

The value of Section 2(5) of the Act has also been established beyond question. The absence of any overt authority in law for the former statutory bodies to provide advice to their practitioners undoubtedly handicapped them. The authority with which the new Council was endowed was extremely important and has been well used.

The Code of Professional Conduct for the Nurse, Midwife and Health Visitor made a major impact on practice. So also have the other advisory documents issued by the Council. The release of these advisory documents has proved to have a value far beyond their contents and the information and challenge they have conveyed. They have contributed to opening channels of communication between the Council and those on its register. Now the Council communicates regularly (through its directly mailed publication *Register*) with practitioners at least twice in each year. For their part many of those practitioners feel no hesitation about communicating with the Council to air and share the dilemmas they face in the course of their professional practice. This has been a most healthy development.

STRUCTURAL PROBLEMS

One of the less satisfactory aspects of the Act has proved to be that which required a significant overlap between the membership of the Council and the National Boards. The resultant problems have nothing whatever to do with the attitudes or willingness of the 28 Council members who are also members of one or another of the National Boards. It results from the impossibility of giving adequate time and attention to each of those organisations while at the same time satisfying the requirements of the employing authority which pays their salary.

No doubt a structure with this kind of overlapping membership appealed to the policy makers and parliamentary draughtsmen in the years 1977 to 1979. The concept of a system for the determination of educational policy which is known to be acceptable to those who have to carry it into action is appealing. It falters, however, if a substantial number of members are unable to give to the work the time it requires and committees have to be cancelled for lack of a quorum.

A Government-commissioned study by management consultants Peat Marwick McLintock, the report of which was submitted to ministers in 1989, identified the problems resulting from the present overlapping membership and recommended that it be brought to an end. Those consultants also recommended an end to the arrangements whereby the role of investigating allegations of misconduct lies with the National Boards. Those changes cannot be achieved without amendment of the Act.

PROFESSIONAL CONDUCT COMMITTEE DELAYS

When I wrote the first edition of *Professional Discipline in Nursing* in 1981 I indicated that the Disciplinary Committee of the General Nursing Council for England and Wales was then meeting for three full days each month and emphasised the burden that this was imposing on the pool of members from which that committee was convened. How light that workload now seems, viewed in retrospect and with knowledge of the UKCC Professional Conduct Committee workload just nine years later.

As 1990 draws to a close the Professional Conduct Committee was meeting for 16 full days each month, yet still the backlog of cases waiting to be heard and the associated elapse time since the original complaint is disturbingly long. In addition, some of the same members had to serve on the Health Committee for two days of meetings each month, all this being in addition to full Council meetings, other committees concerned with such matters as educational policy, midwifery, health visiting, registration and ethics, National Board commitments (for 28 of the 45 members) and salaried employment. So why is there such a delay and backlog? There are a number of reasons.

First, there is the sheer volume of cases. There are more than 600 000 people with currently effective registration on the UKCC's register. There are many more whose names are on the register but whose registration is not currently effective for the purposes of practice. All these people can become the subject of complaints alleging misconduct (some following criminal convictions) in the manner described in Chapter 6. It only needs a very small percentage of this registered population to become the subject of complaint for the Investigating Committees and Professional Conduct Committee to have a very heavy workload that must be performed in the public interest.

The type of cases

Next is the type of cases that make up the caseload with which the committees are faced. When I prepared the previous edition of this book in 1981 I drew upon the statistical information available from the then existing General Nursing Council for England and Wales. It revealed that more than two-thirds of the cases being considered by that Council's Disciplinary Committee were true conviction cases. That is to say that guilt on which the alleged misconduct was based had already been established in criminal courts and that this formed the basis on which the committee proceeded. The figures reveal that, in 1979–1980, the Disciplinary Committee was hearing an average of over five new cases each committee day.

This is no longer the case. Now the true conviction cases form a minority of those referred for hearing by the Professional Conduct Committee and allegation cases a substantial majority. More cases in which direct evidence has to be given by witnesses in public and under oath inevitably means that much more time is consumed. In the statistical year 1989–1990 the Professional Conduct Committee of the UKCC heard an average of only 1.3 new cases each committee day.

The origin of cases

A number of other points need to be made about the composition of the Professional Conduct Committee caseload. It is no surprise that, as the members of the public become better informed (either about how the professions are regulated or about how to find such information) and more aware of their rights, more allegation cases come from that source. Nor should it be regarded as surprising that the publication and distribution of the Code of Professional Conduct, replete as it is with challenge to practitioners to recognise and address the primacy of the interests of patients and clients, has led to an increase in the number of cases that result from colleague complaints. The view formally held by many practitioners that, if you saw a colleague dabbling with drugs or treating a frail patient in a harsh and unkind manner, that was nothing to do with you seems to have been steadily fading. Inappropriate loyalty to colleagues is being replaced by appropriate action on behalf of patients. The cases that emanate from these two sources, unless the allegations are admitted, involve evidence which, with cross-examination and committee questioning, inevitably takes quite a lot of time.

The rules of procedure

Another contributory factor to the increased amount of time the average case consumes is to be found in the statutory rules that now govern the procedures of the committee. By comparison with the comparable procedural rules of the previous committees on which the law conferred the power to remove practitioners from their respective professional registers, the rules now applying compare more closely with those applying in criminal courts and must therefore be seen as more respectful of the principles of justice. This also adds to the elapse time of a hearing, but rightly so since the ultimate sanction available to the committee is so great.

Possibly inappropriate referrals

All of that being said, it has to be conceded that, although referral to the Professional Conduct Committee of any case is intended to be '. . . with a view to removal from the register . . .', less than half of the cases have been concluding in that way. This fact led the UKCC, in 1990, to prepare and release the new advisory document which is reproduced in Appendix 1.

Problems in convening Professional Conduct Committees

Under the heading 'Structural Problems' above, reference has been made to the burdens on members within the present structure. These burdens are reflected in the difficulties experienced in assembling Professional Conduct Committees with sufficient frequency to first erode the backlog of referred cases and then maintain that improved position. No one is in any doubt that the public is not receiving the protection it requires and deserves if a hearing of charges that may result in removal of a practitioner from the register only takes place 2 years after the events giving rise to those changes. The entire professional regulatory system is at risk of becoming discredited unless this problem can be resolved.

The number of Professional Conduct Committee meetings

As can be seen the UKCC has addressed the problem of delay in a number of ways. It has done so by the steady increase in the number of hearing days. It is now often the case that two Professional Conduct Committees will be meeting in different venues on the same day. It has issued the advisory document which it is hoped will control the flow of cases and help to make it possible to hear very quickly those cases which need to be resolved as an urgent matter of public protection.

A defect in the Act

The UKCC has identified a defect in the Nurses, Midwives and Health Visitors

Act 1979 and resolved that an amendment be sought as soon as a bill to amend the Act is in prospect.

That which has, in the light of considerable experience, been identified as a defect is to be found in Section 12(3) of the Act. Referring to the committees which have the power to remove persons from the register (i.e. determined by current statutory rules as the Professional Conduct Committee and the Health Committee), this section states that:

> 'The Committees shall be constituted from members of the Council; and the rules shall so provide that the members of a committee constituted to adjudicate upon the conduct of any person are selected with due regard to the professional field in which that person works.'

I feel sure that the reader will readily see the good sense of the latter part of Section 12(3). It would not be appropriate to have a case concerning a practising midwife heard by a committee without midwife members. The same point can be applied irrespective of the speciality from which the respondent comes. If, however, the respondent works in a speciality from which the Council has no members it becomes impossible to honour the 'due regard' requirement of the Act. The best alternative, recognising its limitations, is to call one or more expert witnesses from the speciality concerned to help the committee members become aware of key practice-related issues.

Possible solutions

This problem could only be resolved in one of two ways. Either the size of the Council could be enormously increased and places guaranteed for a wide range of identified specialities. Such a change would increase the cost of professional regulation which is wholly met by fees paid by the professions' practitioners and would not bring any benefits to other areas of the Council's work. Alternatively Section 12(3) of the Act could be amended so as to allow the two committees concerned to include some members who are not members of the Council. The only Council committees for which this is not permissible under existing law are those empowered to remove persons from the register.

The UKCC declared its support for the latter course in the early part of 1987 and indicated that it wished to see an amendment which would enable it, while continuing to use a committee of five people, to use three Council members and two others from the practising profession.

Spreading the load – increasing the benefits

The use of non-Council members, either in isolation or together with cessation of overlapping Council and Board membership, would, by spreading the enormous burden of this important area of work more widely, make it possible to hold more frequent meetings and erode the backlog of cases. It would appear to have obvious benefits for the public. This change would also prove beneficial for those respondents who, when the evidence is heard, are found not guilty but who have had to wait a long time to clear their names of the allegations made and for witnesses whose memories would have had less opportunity to fade.

There would be other significant benefits. If committee members are drawn from a larger pool it will inevitably involve more people in direct clinical practice.

This should result in a truer form of peer judgment. It would also involve more people in such hearings, who would find in them (as existing Council members do) important messages and lessons to bear back to their own workplaces.

Supplementary member selection

When the time comes for such a change to come into operation it would now be relatively easy, using the Council's computerised register and the evidence it provides of those with currently effective registration, to randomly select a supplementary pool of people who were identified as eligible to serve for up to a maximum number of days in a fixed period of 1 or 2 years. The selection would ensure a geographical spread, a broad age mix and a wide range of specialities. Those identified could then be provided with a study pack and arrangements made for them to attend training sessions and observe the Professional Conduct Committee in action before their period of eligibility began.

As with periods of eligibility for jury service, some identified as eligible may not be called if the nature of the cases in the period does not so require. The process of preparation would still be professionally beneficial. I believe that the profession is ready for such a change and would benefit from it. It is good to see that the management consultants (Peat Marwick McLintock) who conducted the Government-commissioned review of the Council and National Boards (and thus of the working of the Nurses, Midwives and Health Visitors Act 1979) adopted this proposal and recommended such a change in its report.

SUSPENSION FROM PRACTICE

The Nurses, Midwives and Health Visitors Act 1979 provided for the continuation of the power (to be used selectively) to suspend a midwife from practice if that midwife is the subject of a report to the statutory bodies which might possibly culminate in removal from the register. In the previous edition of this book I expressed surprise that the power had not been extended by the Nurses, Midwives and Health Visitors Act 1979 to apply, in limited and justifiable circumstances, to nurses and health visitors. The absence of such a power, particularly at a time when the elapse time between an original complaint and the Professional Conduct Committee hearing has been long, must inevitably have left the public at risk for many months from practitioners who were eventually removed from the register.

THE CASE FOR A CONSUMER VOICE

Given the wording of Section 12(3) of the Nurses, Midwives and Health Visitors Act 1979, it can be seen that the only people who are not nurses, midwives and health visitors who can serve on the Professional Conduct Committee are the few who are Council members.

Existing 'lay' membership

The 'lay' Council members, appointed to Council membership by the Secretary of State under the terms of Section 1(4) of the Act, in order to satisfy those terms are '... registered medical practitioners, or have such qualifications and experience in education or other fields as, in the Secretary of State's opinion, will be of value to the Council in the performance of its functions.' In other words, those members who are not nurses, midwives or health visitors are not really appointed to bring a consumer voice to bear in the Council's decision making but for the medical, educational, financial and management knowledge and expertise they bring.

The small number of members appointed in this way who are not registered medical practitioners and who, although appointed for other reasons, might be regarded as bringing a consumer view, are insufficient in number (five only) to even make it possible for one to participate in every Professional Conduct Committee hearing. In this respect the UKCC is unlike the General Medical Council which is required to have a lay member presence in every Professional Conduct Committee convened. Jean Robinson, in her publication 'A patient voice at the GMC – A lay member's view of the General Medical Council'[2] writes favourably about the manner in which the UKCC fulfils its regulatory functions. She is, however, critical of the fact that there is no requirement to have a consumer member or members on any Professional Conduct Committee, though she recognises that the fault is with the law rather than the way in which that law is operated.

Improved consumer participation

It may well be that, if this problem is to be addressed, it also could be resolved by a method similar to that suggested for enlarging the professional practitioner pool for Professional Conduct Committees rather than by a significant inrease in the Council membership. It is assumed that the official community bodies such as the Association of Community Health Councils would be willing to cooperate in identifying suitable participant members if Parliament decides to legislate for such a change.

THE SINGLE HEARING

Under the former professional disciplinary arrangements it was possible for one person who was both a nurse and a midwife and who was registered with the relevant bodies for England/Wales, Scotland and Northern Ireland to be the subject of five disciplinary hearings as a result of one alleged misdemeanour. Although that was extremely rare, two or three hearings before different statutory bodies was not uncommon. On occasion the decisions were not consistent.

One distinct advantage of the present system is that one hearing only need take place by one Professional Conduct Committee equipped to consider the person in respect of all parts of the register on which his or her name appears. The importance of the 'due regard' point is emphasised by the nature of the task faced by such a committee.

THE HEALTH COMMITTEE RANGE OF DECISIONS

It has been explained that the Nurses, Midwives and Health Visitors Act 1979 made it possible (under that 'or otherwise' phrase in Section 12(1)(a)), to establish the means of protecting the public from the persons whose fitness to practise is seriously impaired by illness. This power was welcomed and has been used to good effect.

Unfortunately the very passage that contains that helpful phrase contains other words which have proved unhelpful. I remind you that Section 12 requires the Council to, by statutory rules, '. . . determine circumstances in which and the means by which a person may, for misconduct or otherwise, be removed from the register. . .'.

The case for 'suspension'

In preparing the draft rules concerning the establishment of the Panel of Screeners, the Health Committee and their procedures and range of decisions, the Council took the view that different terminology should be used in respect of the person prevented from practising by a Health Committee than for the person prevented from practising as a registered practitioner by the Professional Conduct Committee.

In other words, although it believed it appropriate to use the term 'removal from the register' where misconduct in a professional sense had been proved, the Council was of the view that a less stigmatising word such as 'suspended' would be appropriate where the Health Committee found a person unfit to practise due to illness. This was not permitted, however, by the Government Law Officers who have to approve the rules made under Section 12 of the Act, since it would fall outside the powers of the Act which allows only for a person to be 'removed'. It is to be hoped that this differentiation might be made possible by a future change in primary legislation.

MAINTAINING COMPETENCE

The Nurses, Midwives and Health Visitors Act 1979 makes improvement in standards of professional conduct both a mandatory requirement and a principal function of the UKCC. It also empowers that Council to give advice to nurses, midwives and health visitors on standards of conduct.

Clause 3 of the Code of Professional Conduct

In responding to that requirement and using that power the Council has, through its Code of Professional Conduct for the Nurse, Midwife and Health Visitor, made the maintenance and improvement of professional knowledge and competence a matter of 'conduct' which must be addressed in the exercise of personal professional accountability.

It can be seen from the pages of this book that, for all its present imperfections in operation, the UKCC has the power and means to protect the vulnerable public from the practitioner deemed guilty of some culpable action or omission called misconduct by removing him or her from the professional register. It can also be seen that it has the power to protect the public from the practitioner whose fitness to practise is seriously impaired by illness. What the Council has not been equipped to do is to protect the public from the practitioner who is intractably incompetent.

Post-registration education and practice

The problem of incompetence is being addressed through the Council's *Post-Registration Education and Practice Project Report*[3] which is the subject of wide consultation at the time that this manuscript is completed. It is to be hoped that the vast majority of practitioners will respond in a positive and enthusiastic manner to the arrangements for maintaining and improving competence that result. If the gap in the arrangements for the protection of the public is to be made complete it will be necessary, however, for procedures under the law to be developed to consider the position of the person who cannot or will not achieve a competence relevant to the role as a practitioner they are seeking to fill.

CONCLUSION

In this chapter I have endeavoured to review certain aspects of the Nurses, Midwives and Health Visitors Act 1979 and to give a personal view of that piece of primary law in operation. I have commented in particular on those parts of the Act which are germaine to the main subject areas of this book.

The reader can probably detect that, on balance, I feel that the Act has brought many advantages to set against only a few disadvantages. I believe that to be the case, as I do that fairly modest amendments to the Act could turn it into a far more effective instrument for the protection of the public.

REFERENCES

[1] *Project 2000 – A new preparation for practice.* London: UKCC, 1986.
[2] Robinson J. (1988) A patient voice at the GMC – a lay member's view of the General Medical Council. London: *Health Rights*.
[3] *Post-Registration Education and Practice Project Report.* London: UKCC, 1990.

Chapter 11

Looking to the Future

In this book I have endeavoured to do a number of things all at once. Although, on the face of it, some of the subjects covered may be regarded as separate and each possibly deserving more substantial coverage in its own right, I maintain that it is appropriate to address them to the degree I have in one volume.

PROFESSIONAL REGULATION

I have referred, in Chapters 3, 4 and 10 to the law which is concerned with the regulation of the profession. I trust that what I have written there and elsewhere in these pages has conveyed the correct impression that I am a strong advocate of professional self-regulation. For me, one of the hallmarks of any profession is that it accepts the responsibility of regulating itself in the public interest, determines to do it well and strives constantly to review critically and revise its procedures to ensure that these objectives are met.

Professional regulation involves the maintenance and use of the professional register, control over admission to the register, advice and assistance to those whose names are on the register and (where necessary) removal from the register. The register should not be regarded as simply a huge list of names kept by a bureaucratic organisation, but as a source of information for both the public and employers to indicate exactly who the people are from whom an appropriate level of both competence and conduct may be expected.

It needs to be recognised, however, that this professional self-regulation in which I invest such faith is a delicate flower which, unless nurtured, will fade. It is therefore essential that we do it well, or we shall find that the privilege and associated responsibility is taken from us. That, I am convinced, would prove to be contrary to the public interest.

PROFESSION, PROFESSIONAL RESPONSIBILITY AND PROFESSIONAL ACCOUNTABILITY

In Chapters 1 and 2 I have sought to explore the concept of profession and of professional responsibility. In Chapters 5 and 9 I have taken that further by elaborating upon the new challenges that have emerged from the profession's new regulatory body since July 1983. This has, I hope, focused attention upon changes in attitude and activity which have done much to justify (for the nursing, midwifery and health visiting professions) self-regulation status and keep the ground fairly firm at a time when the professions generally have been faced with unprecedented challenges to their authority.

REMOVAL FROM THE REGISTER

In Chapters 6 and 7 and Appendix 1 I have explained the present system which operates to consider allegations that certain practitioners may need to be removed from the professional Register, not as any form of punishment but because the interests of patients and clients so requires. Chapter 12 provides a set of case studies illustrating this important area of work which can be used to facilitate further study.

CARING FOR COLLEAGUES

In Chapter 8 I have described an important means by which the profession demonstrates concern for those removed or at risk of removal from the Register and seeks to assist their recovery and rehabilitation.

WHERE ARE THE PROBLEMS?

Chapters 9 and 10 contain my attempts to review how things stand. That is to say I have commented fairly critically upon the faults of some practitioners, some managers, some employers and some aspects of the existing law in order that those faults may be addressed.

Throughout the period of time that I have been preparing this text I have been mindful of the fact that the environment within which practitioners of nursing, midwifery and health visiting are practising and seeking to deliver a high standard of care and treatment to their patients and clients is often far from satisfactory and sometimes overtly hostile. With something of a wry smile, and recognising that it still holds good today I have noticed that, in the 'Prologue' to her *Notes on Nursing* (first published in 1859), Florence Nightingale wrote that:

> Bad sanitary, bad architectural and bad administrative arrangements often make it impossible to nurse.[1]

I do not refer to this 19th Century statement and its continuing relevance in order to offer to nurses, midwives and health visitors an excuse for any failure to achieve high standards. Florence Nightingale drew attention to it in the prologue to her book in order to go on to attempt to provide a solution for the problems she had identified. I believe that the Code of Professional Conduct and the UKCC's other advice does much the same thing. The response to that challenge cannot come only from the Council, but must largely be composed of the personal actions of each and every person on its register.

It is my contention, therefore, that all the issues that I have covered – profession, professional self-regulation, professional discipline, fitness, competence, accountability, the register – come together as being concerned with serving the interests of the vulnerable public, to whom I have dedicated this book.

INHERITANCE

For several years now I have had a small poster on the wall of my office. Its original intention was to present an ecological message – something that I believe it does extremely well. For me, however, and many visitors to my office from the

United Kingdom and overseas, it has had the additional benefit of conveying an important professional message. The words on the poster are:

We do not inherit the world from our parents. We borrow it from our children.

In professional terms it is saying to us, is it not, that while we owe a great deal to our professional predecessors who fought to achieve the regulatory structure that we are prone to take for granted, we owe still more to our successors in the professions of nursing, midwifery and health visiting. We owe it to them to hand on a profession in good order and a sound professional regulatory structure, not for the sake of the profession itself, but for the sake of the people it exists to serve.

I refer, of course, to a profession that promotes what is good and opposes what is bad; a profession that continues to respond to the increasing technical demands made of it yet without forsaking those essential qualities of care, kindness, compassion and honesty; a profession made up of people who are professionals in their own right and conscious of the responsibilities that they bear for standards; a profession which bases its practice on sound ethical principles. I hope that this book assists to that end.

REFERENCE

1 Nightingale F. (1859) *Notes on Nursing*. Republished in 1980. Edinburgh: Churchill Livingstone.

Chapter 12

Professional Conduct Committee Case Studies: 'Could This Happen Where You Work?'

(To be considered in association with Chapters 6 and 8)

By now the reader should have a reasonable understanding of the way in which the nursing, midwifery and health visiting profession uses the Professional Conduct Committee as an important part of its regulatory process. For the individual or group wishing to go further into the subject and to stimulate group discussion a number of case studies are set out in this chapter.

These case studies are based directly on actual cases considered by the Professional Conduct Committee in the period 1986 to 1990. They are in précis form since they reduce to a few paragraphs of text what emerged before the committee over several hours or even days. They ask you to adopt the role of a Professional Conduct Committee member.

The decisions made by the committee in these cases, together with some comments, are provided in Appendix 4. I suggest that reference be made to that section only after each case has been read, considered and discussed.

CASE A1

A 31-year-old midwife appeared before the Professional Conduct Committee to answer charges of misconduct arising out of incidents which occurred in a labour ward when she was in charge on night duty.

In particular she was alleged to be guilty of misconduct for having, while attending a patient in labour, failed to take appropriate action when the cardiotocographic trace was suggestive of fetal distress or when meconium was noted in the patient's liquor, failed to seek medical advice regarding the above, and allowed the patient to continue expulsive efforts for too long. As a procedural ploy (through the solicitor representing her on behalf of her professional organisation) she denied the facts alleged (though accepting their essential accuracy) in order that the full evidence should be before the committee at the time it considered the contention that, taken in their disturbing context, and notwithstanding the tragic outcome, those facts should not be regarded as misconduct in a professional sense.

The patient concerned had been admitted in spontaneous labour at 8.15 AM on the day preceding the night in question, six days before the estimated date of delivery of a second child. Given the basis on which the case was being fought (i.e. that the denial was technical and that the real issues was whether the facts did or did not amount to misconduct in a professional sense) it was particularly important to be clear about the relationship between needs and resources at various stages of the night and the roles of some other practitioners and how they had conducted themselves.

The labour ward consisted of three delivery rooms, a single side room, a double side room, and a ward to accommodate six. On the night in question the staff at the commencement of the night shift was the respondent with one other midwifery sister and two student midwives (both two months into training). The charges related to the period from about 5.30 AM onwards.

At 9.00 PM (when the night staff came on) there were three patients in established labour (one with a known intrauterine death) and four patients in the six-bedded ward who had been given Prostin pessaries earlier in the evening. There were therefore seven patients and four staff (two of whom were student midwives).

By 10.00 PM there had been two admissions, and an additional staff midwife had been provided at the respondent's request. There were now four patients in established labour (the patient with the intrauterine death being in the single room), one patient seemingly on the verge of a pre-term labour and the four patients who had been given the Prostin.

By 11.00 PM the threatened pre-term labour (26 weeks) had become a reality.

At 00.30 AM another staff midwife arrived to help cover for meal breaks making the situation nine patients and five staff (including the two student midwives), but this was immediately offset by staff being sent for breaks to help ensure availability for the likely high workload later in the night.

At 1.00 AM another patient was admitted in labour and joined the patient in the double room. There were now ten patients and a staff temporarily reduced to two. At 1.30 AM the staff numbers restored to five, after which the respondent took her break.

At 3.00 AM there were ten patients of whom five were in established labour and the staff was again five (including the students). The patient who was identified in the charges had been in a delivery room all night. The intrauterine death patient was in the single room with her husband. The respondent was dividing her time between these two patients as well as performing her supervisory duties.

At 3.30 AM the respondent called a doctor as her delivery room patient was pyrexial. Some antibiotics were prescribed. The nursing officer called shortly after that, and confirmed in evidence that she looked at the patient's CTG trace and considered it satisfactory.

At 5.15 AM the intrauterine death patient eventually delivered. This sad delivery was complicated by a broken cord, and the placenta was retained, then being delivered by the respondent with maternal effort. The nature and significance of the time spent by the respondent with these parents was reflected in a letter from them submitted in the latter part of the case which expressed thanks for the support and kindness shown in and around the delivery, and telling her they had felt able to accept a photograph of the baby to keep and would be attending her funeral.

At 5.50 AM the respondent telephoned the nursing officer to report the delivery of the dead baby, and also asked for assistance from another midwife. She was sent an auxiliary.

There were now ten patients and six staff, only three of whom were midwives. The need for appropriate staff grew when, following conversations with two ladies who telephoned from their homes at about 6.00 AM, those patients arrived in the unit shortly before 7.00 AM.. There were now 12 patients and the same six staff. The respondent was also having to give more time to the patient admitted in labour at 1.00 AM.

It was during this period from 5.30 AM onwards that the trace on the baby identified in the charges on two occasions went down to 60 beats per minute, then rising to 160 and by 6.15 AM to above 180. It was contended that when the respondent next saw the trace after a dip to 60 a doctor should have been called, and even more when the dips persisted and became more frequent in the period from 6.40 AM to 7.45 AM. The staff midwife had briefly gone into the room at 7.00 AM, noted the deceleration on the trace, but also noted the recovery.

At 7.45 AM the respondent entered the delivery room with the midwife who was to relieve the student. She looked at the fetal heart trace and immediately saw the significance of the huge decelerations which had failed to register with her as she earlier came in and out. A crash call was put out and an emergency forceps delivery was performed, but unfortunately the infant was stillborn.

It is now necessary to refer to the nursing officer and the other midwifery sister and to how they perceived and performed their roles. The nursing officer emerged as a person whose managerial style might most politely be described as non-interventionist, since she clearly stated that though she had responsibility for the organisation and disposition of staff she would not offer assistance unless she first received a request. As for the other midwifery sister, she appeared to the committee as someone who was determined to do no more than she had to, and to work at her own pace. She had been undertaking a delivery with the second student, and did the post-delivery work in an unhurried way, resisting the respondent's requests that she hurry and become involved in either admitting one of the new patients or relieve the respondent with one of her patients.

In her own evidence the respondent (who had been a midwifery sister for four years in two hospitals at the time of the incident) stated from the study of the tracings placed before her that the latest time when it was likely to prove possible to safely deliver the baby was 5.30 AM, and that it was an error in her practice to allow the labour to progress until 7.45 AM. She stated that no blame should be attached to the student since she was an extra pair of eyes and ears for the respondent and not in a decision-making role. She said the responsibility was entirely her own. She added that with hindsight the fetal heart trace was obviously disturbing and that she could only say that she was so taken up with her own allocation of patients as well as the general pressure of work that she failed to recognise the significance of what she was seeing.

It also emerged in evidence that this level of staffing relative to workload was not unusual. The respondent stated that she did not make further representations when sent the auxilliary as she was so used to it happening. With a number of colleagues she had (four months earlier) written to the District Nursing Officer to draw attention to the pressure of the workload and the resultant low morale in the midwifery unit.

In spite of the representations made on behalf of the respondent the committee found the facts to be misconduct in a professional sense. Do you agree?

At the mitigation/aggravation stage the director of midwifery services for the health authority made it clear that the respondent was a highly motivated, knowledgeable, competent and respected practitioner. Subsequent to registration as a nurse and midwife she had undertaken a specialised course in labour ward intensive care. One year before these incidents she had successfully completed an Advanced Diploma in Midwifery, and was accepted to study for a Midwives Teachers Diploma had the incidents not occurred. She still supported the respondent's aspirations to undertake those studies. The committee also received an impressive number of letters of support from former colleagues.

Given that the facts were proved and considered to be misconduct, what judgment would you then pass on this midwife? Would you postpone judgment, remove from the register, or take no action except possibly to utter some cautionary or advisory words?

In addition, what (if any) recommendations would you make to the health authority, and what lessons does the case contain that might be applied where you work?

CASE A2

A registered nurse for the mentally handicapped appeared before the Professional Conduct Committee to answer allegations of misconduct arising out of incidents alleged to have occurred during and in association with a holiday for some residents of the hospital in which he was employed as a staff nurse. The nurse had been registered for two years at the time that he was dismissed from employment and made the subject of the allegations which called into question his registration status.

The nurse had been approached by his superiors and asked if he would take eight mentally handicapped residents on holiday to a seaside location approximately 200 miles away from the hospital. The residents were from a ward other than that on which he worked as a staff nurse and were not known to him. He would be accompanied by a nursing assistant from the ward which housed those residents. He agreed to do as requested and arranged several visits to the appropriate ward to meet the said residents and learn something of their behaviour, medicine regimes, etc. He was not involved in preparing the container of medicines which was to be taken on holiday, that responsibility being in the hands of the sister of the ward.

At an early hour on a Saturday morning he collected the hospital minibus (for which he was to be the only driver) and then went to the ward to collect his nursing assistant colleague, the residents who were to participate in the holiday and the necessary equipment including the assembled box of medicines. In respect of the medicines, he was simply accepting the word of the sister that the contents were in order and satisfied the prescriptions for the residents which were also said to be enclosed in the box.

The holiday for the residents apparently went extremely well and gave no cause for complaint. The respondent nurse found, however, on only day 2 of the 7-day holiday, that while the medicine box contained the necessary medicines to respond to all regular prescriptions, those to be administered only on an 'as required' basis had not been included. Faced with this situation and a need being manifested by two of the residents, rather than telephone the hospital to seek assistance, the nurse took them to a general practitioner, explained the situation, and was given prescriptions for the missing 'as required' medicines which he then obtained from a retail chemist and used as appropriate.

So successful was the holiday in modifying (for the better) the behaviour of several of the residents who normally demonstrated disturbed behaviour that the respondent nurse, exercising his personal professional judgment, decided that, since their change of environment and activity had significantly modified their behaviour, they need not be given all of their behaviour modifying medicines. He did not seek authority by telephone from the hospital for this change in regime.

At the end of a successful week he, with his nursing assistant colleague, assisted the residents to pack their property into the hospital minibus, packed and locked the medicine container, paid a final visit to the beach with the residents and then began his long drive back to the hospital. He encountered heavy traffic and significant delays on some stretches of road and this, together with essential breaks, resulted in him reaching the hospital quite late in the evening and in a very tired state. He returned the patients to their ward and handed the medicine box and keys to the sister, indicating at the same time that although he was now officially on holiday he would return two days later to complete his reports and deal with any residual matters. He then went to his own home feeling that, although it had been a hard week, he had done a difficult job fairly well and could feel reasonably satisfied.

Two days later he interrupted his period of leave to go to the hospital and in particular to the ward which accommodated the residents to complete his report work and deal with any residual documentation. On reaching the ward he was shocked to be steered immediately into a side room and kept there while a senior nurse manager was called. On arrival the manager told him that he was not to be permitted to enter that ward or indeed his own ward because he was suspended from duty on full pay while an investigation was conducted into discrepancies in the contents of the medicine container. He was provided with no opportunity to explain the situation, nor was he asked questions that might have elicited information that was relevant to such an enquiry but was sent home to wait to be called for an investigatory hearing.

Eventually, following an investigation conducted to the apparent satisfaction of the hospital managers, a disciplinary hearing took place and the respondent nurse was both dismissed from employment and made the subject of allegations of misconduct which eventually became the subject of a hearing before the Professional Conduct Committee. The allegations he faced were (1) that he had behaved improperly and unnecessarily by obtaining prescriptions from a general practitioner rather than calling the hospital and (2) that he had withheld prescribed medicines from mentally handicapped residents.

At the hearing before the Professional Conduct Committee it emerged clearly in evidence that the contents of the medicine box (which had been packed by other nurses more senior than himself and with knowledge of the residents) had not included the 'as required' medicines even though records demonstrated that they were required in the ward setting from time to time. It also emerged that, rather than have their behaviour adversely affected by the withholding of prescribed behaviour modifying medicines, the behaviour of the residents in their small holiday hotel and in various places of entertainment to which they had been taken had been exemplary. It appeared that, in many respects, the respondent nurse was being criticised for adopting a more flexible approach than that which would have been the norm for those who brought the complaints against him and for his willingness to exercise his personal judgment in the circumstances in which he found himself.

The nurse was not denying at all that the box which he returned contained some medicines which had not been there when he left or that it contained a larger quantity of some other medicines than would have been the case if those medicines had been administered directly in accordance with the prescription charts. He concentrated instead on explaining why this was the case and justifying his actions. It was not, therefore, a matter of difficulty to establish the facts set out at the beginning of this paragraph. He sought to persuade the Committee that those facts did not constitute misconduct in a professional sense since they were the product of actions taken in the interests of the residents in his care at a time when he was the only specialist nurse present, having been given the burden of responsibility by senior nurses who presumably believed him appropriate to bear that burden.

Place yourself in the position of the members of the Professional Conduct Committee. Given this set of circumstances how would you have voted when required to determine whether these facts constitute misconduct in a professional sense? If you say it is not misconduct the case closes. If you say that it is misconduct you will need to proceed and determine whether to postpone judgment, remove this nurse from the register or simply administer some words of caution and counsel. Irrespective of your decisions on the above points, consider also what representations you would wish to be made to the Chairman of the Health Authority or its managers about the facts that had emerged in evidence.

CASE A3

A very experienced midwife appeared before the Professional Conduct Committee as a result of incidents alleged to have occurred following the admission to an antenatal ward of a young woman at 29 weeks gestation suffering from an antepartum haemorrhage. The particular allegations were:

(1) that she performed a vaginal examination when it was contraindicated;
(2) that she administered a drug (namely Yutopar) intravenously without a written prescription or other authority from a doctor;
(3) that she knew or ought to have known that the drug was contraindicated by the patient's condition (it is a drug to delay premature labour but which is contraindicated in antepartum haemorrhage);
(4) that she administered the said drug without checking it with another trained person as the local policy required;
(5) that she falsely marked the patient's fluid and drug additives chart to indicate that the drug had been checked by the labour ward sister; and
(6) that she had failed to label the infusion bag with details of its contents as the local policy and good practice required.

The respondent midwife was present and represented by a barrister instructed by a professional organisation. The charges were denied.

Evidence in support of the charges came from a doctor (the senior house officer in obstetrics) and the labour ward sister. The doctor indicated that, in response to a GP's call indicating that a patient had experienced a small blood loss 'per vagina' he had arranged for her admission. When she had been admitted by the respondent he came to see her. He stated that he found her well with no further blood loss. He noticed that the midwife's notes indicated that she had performed a vaginal examination and was surprised as it was contraindicated in the condition, but did not comment. He stated that he wrote up his admission notes, but was then called to the operating theatre to assist with an emergency Caesarian section. He indicated that on his return he would 'put up a plain drip' to keep a vein open in anticipation of some more significant bleeding, and asked that it be prepared. He had not at this stage formally prescribed anything or verbally requested that any IV additives be prepared. Following the operation he returned to the ward, inserted the canula and connected the prepared infusion. He said he was shown no chart, but agreed he should have signed for the IV fluid. He insisted that the bag was not labelled to indicate the presence of any IV additives. He further stated that he was telephoned by the staff midwife on night duty 3 hours later at 10.30 PM. She told him that she was concerned to note that the patient admitted with an antepartum haemorrhage that day had an IV infusion up with a normal saline bag labelled to indicate that it contained Yutopar as an additive. He said he told her that was 'a mistake' and that it should be replaced by a 'plain drip'. He did not go to see the patient, stating that the patient's tachycardia was being resolved by stopping the drip with the additive.

The labour ward sister told how the respondent had come to her with an ampoule of Yutopar, asked her to check it, and told her that the doctor had asked that it be prepared for IV infusion to the patient recently admitted with antepartum haemorrhage. She said she told the respondent that it should not be given, that the respondent should firmly tell the doctor why and that if he did not accept it from her to refer him to the labour ward sister. This witness also confirmed that in the 'check by' entry against Yutopar in the IV fluids and additives chart, the entry giving her name was not in her writing.

The documentary evidence submitted included the local policy on IV fluids and additives which contained a clear statement that verbal instructions to administer IV additives must not be acted upon by nursing and midwifery staff.

In response to the allegations the respondent agreed that she had performed 'a very gentle vaginal examination' because she believed from experience that the bleeding might indicate some cervical erosion. She had not used a speculum. She held to the view that the examination was not contraindicated in the circumstances. In respect of the IV infusion and additive, she stated that the doctor had come to the ward when the patient was admitted and saw her briefly. He was then called to the operating theatre, at which time he had not written any notes on the patient or completed any prescription chart or IV fluids/additives chart. As he was about to leave he had told her to prepare for him to put up an IV infusion on his return and to add some Yutopar. She added that she followed him into the corridor and twice questioned the latter instruction but he insisted. She stated that she took an ampoule of Yutopar from the cupboard and went to the labour ward sister with a request that she check it. She took no IV fluids/additives chart because none had been written. She agreed with the evidence given by that witness, but indicated that in spite of the advice received she added the Yutopar to the normal saline bag, labelled it fully with the official adhesive label as the policy required, prepared for the setting up of the IV infusion, and prepared an IV fluids/additives chart by inserting the patient's details, and the normal saline and Yutopar in the appropriate places for the doctor to sign. She gave clear, firm evidence to the effect that, when the doctor returned, she showed him an empty Yutopar ampoule and properly labelled normal saline container, told him the additive had been inserted as requested but again questioned its appropriateness (though not as forcibly as the labour ward sister had urged), that he again stated that was what he wanted and that he then inserted the canula and set up the infusion.

The respondent agreed that she had inserted the name of the labour ward sister in the 'checked by' space on the chart, justifying this by the fact that she had checked the ampoule, and that it was normal practice in this unit (which seemed to be the case). She therefore argued that it had not been done falsely.

The first charge was dependent on whether the Committee thought the vaginal examination was contraindicated, and they did. Do you agree?

Since the infusion bag in question was the first there was considerable argument from the lawyers involved as to whether the midwife or the doctor had 'administered' it. The Committee took a broad view and felt that inserting a drug into the bag (even the first bag) could count as 'administered'. With this technicality out of the way it became a direct conflict of evidence between the respondent and the doctor as to whether he had asked for the drug to be added and whether the bag had been labelled when he put it up.

Certainly it was labelled when the night staff midwife found it and called him, and he had told her it was a 'mistake'. He had not gone to see the patient, or completed the IV fluids/additives chart, or remonstrated with the respondent when she called him to the ward the next day. It was one day later still, when some criticism of the treatment given was emerging, that the doctor went to his consultant and thus a complaint was made leading to the midwife's suspension from practice and report to the statutory bodies.

It came down to a straight issue of credibility, and the members who had questioned both the respondent and the doctor believed the evidence of the former, therefore taking the view that the doctor had made a mistake which he subsequently recognised, and had fabricated a story to protect himself. These two charges and that concerned with 'falsely' entering another name, had to be considered in view of the unsatisfactory practices in the unit. In addition to that concerning the examination, the Committee found proved the charges that she administered a drug which she knew or ought to have known was contraindicated, and that she did so without properly checking with another person.

The committee regarded these three things as misconduct in a professional sense. Do you agree?

At the mitigation/aggravation stage of the hearing the respondent's barrister presented her as a midwife of a generation which did not easily argue with or decline to follow the instruction of a doctor. She had been a registered nurse for 35 years and a midwife for 30 years. Most of her professional life, and certainly the last ten years had been spent in midwifery. Her record (said her manager in profile evidence) had been generally satisfactory, though she had needed more assistance to keep up to date in recent years than most of her colleagues.

What is your judgment on this respondent? You can postpone judgment for a period and set criteria for a resumed hearing, or remove her from the register (as nurse and/or midwife), or give some words of counsel and caution but take no further action.

Ask yourselves whether there are other people who failed to honour their accountability in this setting and comment on their degree of culpability.

In addition consider what lessons emerge which might be applied in your work setting, and what (if any) recommendations you might wish to make to the employing authority.

CASE A4

A community psychiatric nurse appeared before the Professional Conduct Committee charged with misconduct in a professional sense in that he had disclosed confidential information without authority and in breach of his position of trust.

The health authority whose staff this registered mental nurse had joined 18 months before the incident had no inpatient psychiatric care facilities and relied on an adjacent authority to provide a service. Prior to his appointment there had been similar dependence on that authority for a CPN service, but it became clear that one nurse day per week was inadequate. As a result of advertising and interview the nurse who became the respondent in this case was appointed to establish a community psychiatric nursing services.

He was aged 50 years and had entered training when he was 45. Half of his two years post-registered experience had been as a night charge nurse of a psychiatric unit in a district general hospital. He had no experience of nursing in the community or training for the role. On taking up the post he found himself directly responsible to the Assistant Director of Nursing Services for District Nursing and Health Visiting. She was a registered mental nurse but had not had experience of mental nursing for over 20 years. She was not enthusiastic about taking on this additional responsibility when she had less than 2 years to serve before retirement. The respondent found that the need for the service far exceeded the 60 cases he inherited from the former visiting CPNs. His caseload grew fast, and he was soon providing only a crisis intervention service. He complained about this to his managers, and they appointed a second (unqualified) CPN six months after he commenced employment, and a third a further 6 months on. Although the health authority were willing to second the respondent for CPN training, once he had a heavy caseload they could not release him until other staff were in the post. He had only been able to attend a two-day symposium which was an introduction to the role of the CPN.

By the time it was possible for him to take up the training course place a combination of his frustration that it was still a crisis intervention service and the feeling that this was not the role for him led to him allowing one of his colleagues to take the place while he considered a different career plan. The patient about whom it was alleged confidential information had been released was one of the high risk group he received from his colleague to care for (in addition to his own caseload) when that colleague went on the CPN course.

Eighteen months later, when the respondent nurse had left the employment of the health authority and was undertaking a clinical teachers course, the authority received from that patient a writ for damages naming both the authority and the nurse, the claim being based on the allegation that, as a result of the nurse releasing confidential information about him he had lost his employment and had been unable to obtain other employment. After investigating the matter the authority brought the allegations to the statutory bodies, thus calling into question the nurse's registration status and right to practise.

At the Professional Conduct Committee the allegations were denied. There was, however, no dispute about the main facts, but rather about how they were interpreted and the motivation behind the nurse's actions. Note that there were three elements in the charge. That the information disclosed was confidential. That it was disclosed without authority. That this constituted a breach of the nurse's position of trust.

The essential facts were that the patient who originated the writ for damages had made two serious suicide attempts within a three-month period. In the first he deliberately crashed a car into a lamp post, resulting in inpatient treatment of his injuries. The second involved the taking of a substantial quantity of drugs and further inpatient treatment in the general hospital prior to transfer to the adjacent authority's psychiatric inpatient facilities. The psychiatrist from that authority saw him while he was in the general hospital and instructed the respondent to prepare a 'social report'.

This was outside his experience. He used as a model a report prepared by his colleague who was away on the CPN course. He first visited the patient in the general hospital but found him too ill to discuss anything. He visited him again a few days later when he was physically better but extremely hostile and rejected attempts by the nurse to be involved and caring. The respondent did gather, however, that the patient's anger and his attempts on his life had much to do with the fact that his wife had left him (taking the children) and was living with another woman and sharing a lesbian relationship.

The respondent next visited the estranged wife. She told him that her husband was threatening her, her partner and the children with violence. She also stated that he had previous convictions for theft and violence. Being anxious to present a comprehensive and balanced report, the respondent next went to see a person who others had told him was a personal friend of the patient and who had been instrumental in getting him employment on the staff of a college.

Both the respondent and that man agreed in evidence that, having confirmed that the man could be seen in the role of friend as well as the head of the department in which the patient worked, the respondent first told him the estranged wife had spoken of threats of violence and subsequently that she said he had a criminal record which featured violence.

The respondent said that the friend/employer appeared very guarded when told these things which were shared only in order to elicit information about the likely truth or otherwise of the wife's allegations. He added that he had no knowledge as to whether the statement about convictions was true and no means of checking, and was sharing the information with a person he saw as the patient's close friend. The friend/employer said in evidence that he told the respondent that if he was going to make allegations like that he could go away and put them in writing and that nothing would be done about them otherwise. All that the respondent had learnt from him was that the patient had attended a course for the unemployed at the college, had done well, and had been given a staff post teaching basic catering skills to unemployed young people on courses. In spite of his assertion, a few minutes later the man went to the patient (now back at work 'on leave' from the psychiatric hospital to which he was returning at weekends) and told him he had information about a conviction which had not been declared on his job application form which had made it clear that the post was not 'exempt'. The patient indicated that the information about convictions was true, and was asked to resign as the friend/employer could not run the risk of having him on the staff with this background.

The facts being denied, having heard the evidence the committee had to determine whether all the three elements in the charge were proved. Was this confidential information? Was it without authority or consent? (The respondent's representative argued that, being told by the consultant psychiatrist to prepare the report it was assumed he had obtained the necessary consent.) Was it in breach of his position of trust?

See yourself as a member of the committee. What decision do you make, recognising that all three elements have to be proved for the charge to stand? Do you find the charge proved? If you find the charge proved do you consider it misconduct in a professional sense? If 'yes' will you postpone judgment, remove from the register, or close the case with some words of caution or counsel? Consider the adequacy or otherwise of the setting in which it occurred to indicate the comment or criticism you might wish to direct to the managers of the health authority. Consider whether such a thing could happen where you work.

CASE A5

A man aged 32 years, whose qualification was that of a registered nurse for the mentally handicapped (RNMH) appeared before the Professional Conduct Committee to answer a charge that, contrary to the policy of the authority for which he worked he had wrongly and without authority secluded a resident in a small, windowless room without light.

At the hearing, through the full-time officer of the trade union who was representing him, the respondent substantially admitted the allegations whilst arguing that it had been intended as a brief period of secure isolation in the patient's interests, rather than seclusion as that is normally meant.

The key witness in support of the charges was a nursing assistant who came to take over at the beginning of the night shift from the person who was the subject of the case who had been in charge during the second half of the day. She said that, in his departing words as he left the ward, the respondent had said that the patient was 'in the horse-box – let him our when you're ready'. She then set about her work on the ward, where she was alone with approximately 30 mentally handicapped residents (some of them very dependent). The nursing officer came to administer the drugs about 1 hour later, and when he required to give the drugs to the resident in question asked where he was, and was told. With the nursing assistant he then went to release him. He described it as being a large cupboard under the stairs which contained broken beds, etc, but nowhere to sit properly. The evidence of the nursing officer was that the resident seemed unharmed by the experience.

In his defence it was said by and argued for the respondent that he was faced with a difficult situation. The resident in question was often difficult and prone to violence and had been very difficult during the whole of that day, for part of which he had two nursing assistants in support, but for much only one. This had made it necessary to almost 'special' the particular patient, but even then he sought to abscond on several occasions. This was a matter of concern as he had on previous occasions gone to the local village and broken into houses. The respondent did not deny knowledge of the hospital's policy on seclusion, and admitted to knowing that one specific room had been allocated on another ward for any patient for whom seclusion was authorised. That brought the case back repeatedly to the argument that this was not seen as seclusion, but as a temporary isolation in the interest of the patient and others. It was also said that his departing remark had been meant to indicate that the nursing assistant could release the patient as soon as she had taken over the ward.

Some other points seem significant. First, although the patient was said to have been difficult all day, no specific mention had been made in any report. Second, although seemingly having had difficulty with the patient all day when supported by one or two other people, the respondent had not told those in authority that it would not be possible for the one nursing assistant to cope with the situation.

The case was only reported 2½ years after the event, when a new director of nursing arrived, found documentary evidence of the matter, and also found that no local disciplinary action had been taken and no report submitted to the statutory body. Meanwhile the nurse in question had continued employment in the same hospital, though much of the time in a different setting, and had seemingly performed to everybody's satisfaction.

Most of the allegations were admitted. The Committee heard the necessary evidence so as to establish in their minds that they did regard the patient as having been 'secluded'. For the defence it was argued that, seen in context this was not misconduct in a professional sense.

You are now the Professional Conduct Committee. Would you regard the admitted/proven offence as misconduct in a professional sense? If 'yes' would you then decide to postpone judgment, remove from the register, or take no action apart from some words of caution and counsel? Do you have a view on the manner in which previous managers had dealt with the situation? It might be a useful exercise to list the various people who have contributed to this incident.

CASE A6

A 35-year-old district nurse was the subject of a hearing by the Professional Conduct Committee on charges of misconduct arising out of incidents in the course of her work. The hearing was a consequence of the nurse having been convicted in a criminal court of the theft of sums of money from patients she had been visiting in the course of her professional duties.

It emerged from the evidence that the nurse was considered to be caring and skilful. It was also said that she was liked by her patients and formed extremely good relationships with them and any relatives and friends who visited them in their homes at times she was calling. In short, she was liked, respected and above all trusted.

Since the nurse had been convicted in a criminal court and the court had imposed a suspended prison sentence that formed the basis from which the committee had to operate. The official documents certifying the conviction were submitted as proof of the facts alleged. The evidence heard related to the circumstances leading up to those facts.

That evidence indicated that the nurse had a fairly average caseload in terms of numbers, but one that contained an above average number of elderly patients. In the course of her visits to those elderly patients and the need to go to various drawers and cupboards for clothes (etc.) the nurse came to be aware of the places in which some of them were keeping substantial sums of money in bank notes. For example, one had wads of notes in pockets stitched to the sides of her mattress, while another kept them under her clean underclothes in a drawer.

There were six patients involved in the charges. The time came when each of them was either going into hospital as a planned admission or moving house. In each case the nurse volunteered to go (in her own time) to help them pack. It was in the course of this activity that some of the accumulated money was apparently taken. In the case of the five going into hospital, the nurse (writing in her professional capacity rather than as a friend assisting them to pack) wrote notes to accompany them which indicated to the ward staff that the old ladies were confused. Faced with that information the hospital staff had not regarded the matter seriously when the ladies, over their first 2 weeks as inpatients, complained about their lost money. It was only when a relative of one of them did believe the patient and made representations to the district nurse's line manager that the matter was investigated. The details of that investigation need not trouble you, but you need to know that in this way a little over £2000 had been stolen from six elderly, dependent patients.

The facts were established by the certificate of conviction. The Committee then had to determine whether they regarded those facts as misconduct in a professional sense. Look at the Code of Professional Conduct to see what parts of the Council's advice to its practitioners are relevant and then decide whether you would regard those facts as misconduct. The Committee did, and then proceeded to hear evidence as to the previous history of the respondent and any mitigation before retiring to make its decision. '

The respondent had chosen not to attend, not to be represented in her absence and not to submit any mitigation for the consideration of the committee. In order to hear something of her previous history the Committee heard evidence from and questioned her former nursing officer. This witness, speaking from experience over several years and on the basis of monitoring visits done with the respondent, told the committee members that she had always found her to be skilful and competent, with an apparently good relationship with patients and their relatives. She had clearly been shocked by the fact that such allegations had been made and proved against a nurse she had previously believed to be a person of integrity and was distressed at having to give her evidence.

You are now the Professional Conduct Committee. Accepting that the facts have been proved and regarded as misconduct, what is your judgment? Consider also whether any people in this case in addition to the respondent need to be the subject of comment when the Chairman announces the Committee's decision in public, and what lessons emerge for your work setting.

CASE A7

A 30-year-old registered mental nurse appeared before the Professional Conduct Committee as a result of an incident that was alleged to have occurred shortly after he came on duty to commence his shift at 1.30 PM. The charge he faced was to the effect that he had ill-treated a patient by striking her and that he had responded inappropriately to the patient's request for attention.

In the course of the evidence received from the patient and several members of the staff the following picture emerged. The nurse (who became the respondent in this case) had been off duty for the previous two days. On the day in question he came on duty to commence a later shift. He was to be in charge of the ward, it being one of three in a psychiatric unit of a large district general hospital. He received a handover, in the course of which he was made aware that the patient who became involved in the incident (a woman of 50 years of age) had been admitted the previous day with a depressive illness. He recalled that he knew her slightly from an early brief period as an inpatient for the same reason. He was not told of any problems to which she had been seeking to draw attention or of any requests she had made for assistance during the morning and was given no indication to suggest that she had not received (in her view) an appropriate response to her needs and requests.

Having received the handover report the respondent nurse, accompanied by a student nurse, commenced the administration of medicines. They were doing this from the doorway of a small clinical room in which the medicine trolley was securely locked and stored when not in use. The respondent nurse had the trolley located just inside the room and patients were coming to the doorway to receive their prescribed medication. The student was in the clinical room, the respondent nurse and trolley therefore barring his way but not his vision. The nurses' station was located in the corridor and near to the clinical room so that, on emerging from the door of the clinical room it was necessary to deviate slightly to the left to avoid the end of the desk unit.

When prescribed medication was being administered to other patients, the patient in this case came to the trolley (she said in her own evidence that she was fairly angry) and demanded something to treat a headache. She was told by the nurse that there was no appropriate prescription, that she should go away and that he would arrange something for her later. What he did not know (but what became clear from later evidence) was that she had been complaining of a headache and asking to be given something for it during most of the previous shift.

The administration of medicines was nearing completion when the patient returned, vociferously and bluntly complaining of her headache and shouting that she had waited 'all bloody morning' for some tablets. That said, she suddenly thrust a hand towards the containers of medicines in the trolley. The nurse's response to her action was to quickly slam down the lid of the trolley against the patient's hand and lower arm. Her already existing anger being fuelled by this further reaction to her, the patient both generally flailed her arms as if to strike the nurse and produced a stream of expletives indicating what she thought of him. At this stage it was alleged and the evidence indicated that the nurse punched the patient, striking her on the jaw, as a result of which she fell to the floor in the corridor. At that stage he quickly pushed the trolley back into the clinical room and rushed out into the corridor only to crash his thigh against the end of the nurses' station and himself fall to the floor. The evidence indicated that he rose and called the student nurse to assist him and that they together picked the struggling patient up and carried her into the nearest room with beds which ran off the same corridor opposite the clinical room. The intention was to place the struggling patient on the nearest bed, but it transpired that the bed wheels were not locked and as they lent against the bed to do so it ran away from them and the patient again fell to the floor.

The evidence demonstrated that at this point another patient, having shouted the question 'Are you teaching Doris karate?' joined the action by picking up a chair and striking all those involved. Things escalated further with some other patients joining in. In less than two minutes the scene had moved from one patient crossly demanding something for her headache to something approaching a full scale riot. Other staff on the ward and those from other wards in the unit were required to restore order to the scene.

The respondent nurse, while admitting that the patient may have been struck, insisted that it was only a necessary action taken in self-defence as she flailed a series of blows generally in his direction and that he had certainly not punched her on the jaw. This view was contradicted by the evidence of the patient, the student nurse and a domestic assistant who had also witnessed the events.

The facts alleged were therefore denied but were found proved to the standard of proof the law requires (the Committee must be satisfied so that it is sure). That brought the Committee to the stage of the hearing where it must determine whether, when looked at in context, the facts constitute misconduct in a professional sense. What is your decision on that point?

The Committee resolved that the proven facts did constitute misconduct in a professional sense and therefore had to receive any evidence in mitigation and of the previous history of the respondent before making its final judgment on the case. No character evidence was produced by the respondent or his representative. In providing previous history of the respondent a professional manager from the health authority indicated that, in his 2 years of employment with that authority, the respondent had been a generally satisfactory employee, their main concern focusing on the point that he showed little imagination, took no initiatives and was generally reluctant to accept change.

You must now put yourselves in a position of the members of the Professional Conduct Committee and decide on the judgment appropriate to this case which you find it necessary to make, reflecting the profession's global responsibilities to the public. You might also consider what other persons contributed to this incident and their degree of culpability relative to that of the respondent nurse and also ask yourselves whether any particular concerns need to be drawn to the attention of the employing authority as a result of this incident.

CASE A8

A 50-year-old registered general nurse became the subject of charges before the Professional Conduct Committee arising out of matters concerned with the running of the registered nursing home of which she was the proprietor and matron.

The respondent had purchased the property and established a nursing home six years earlier but had decided to sell the nursing home as an operating business. She therefore advertised in appropriate journals and newspapers and as a result was approached by a company engaged in broadcasting which wished to diversify its business interests. A director of the company engaged the services of an experienced nurse to accompany him to view the nursing home.

On that exploratory visit they were generally satisfied with the state of repair of the property and the standards of care that appeared to be provided for the residents though clearly the nurse advisor felt that there were some respects in which there was scope for improvement.

Having decided that this was the type of business in which they wished to invest, the aspiring purchasers engaged a registered nurse to be the matron of the nursing home when purchased, and with her made a further visit to the nursing home with the same general outcome. Having made that visit an offer was made for the purchase of the property as a running business and the offer was accepted.

The new owners settled a date on which they would take over, it being approximately ten weeks from the purchase date. The matron arranged to interview the existing staff of the nursing home with the exception of the proprietor/matron who was moving out. She was not impressed by the staff at the interviews and decided that she would only engage one nursing auxiliary and would advertise and interview to recruit a new team from deputy matron to domestic staff.

On the date fixed for the transfer from old to new management the director involved in the original inspection, together with the newly appointed matron and deputy matron arrived with their staff team at 8 AM on a cold day in winter in accordance with the plans. On entering the home they were immediately struck by the fact that it was very dirty and that there was a strong smell of urine and faeces. They began to walk around the two floors and many rooms of the premises and, to their astonishment, found that the only person present was the one nursing auxiliary the new matron had engaged. It was clearly impossible for her to be providing even vaguely adequate care for the 32 patients accommodated in numerous rooms over two floors. It was also clear that none of the patients had been given breakfast and that no preparations for breakfast were in hand or provisions available.

The new team, in a state of considerable anger, immediately got down to the task of caring for the patients. Their anger rose to new heights as they discovered that one patient after another presented an extremely dirty and unkempt appearance, suggesting that they had received no attention for hours or even possibly days. For example, the skin of some patients over much of their bodies was caked with large quantities of dried faeces that must have been present for a long time. In addition, underneath many of the beds, quantities of fouled incontinence pads had been thrown, it again being clear that they had been there for days.

In continuing the search of the premises the director and matron walked into a small unheated room which, according to the plans and the introduction they had previously been given, was used as a small mortuary for bodies of the deceased prior to the arrival of the undertakers. In this room they found a frail, ill, very old lady in a very dirty and uncared for condition.

The outgoing matron/proprietor was eventually found in her flat at the top of the building, casually packing in preparation for departure. She appeared unmoved by the protests and expressions of concern voiced by the new owner and matron.

In order that independent corroboration could be obtained of the state of affairs at the point of transfer, but without wishing to prolong the neglect of the patients, the new matron asked the appropriate inspecting officers of the relevant health board to attend without delay. They did call about two hours later at which time, in spite of the fact that many patients had been treated and some of the worst contamination removed, they were able to see and record the fact that the condition of the home and its residents was totally unsatisfactory and certainly far worse that at the time of their last formal inspection four months earlier. The new owners, having enquired about their rights in this respect, decided to bring complaints against the outgoing proprietor/matron alleging misconduct in a professional sense.

The charges before the Professional Conduct Committee were to the effect that the matron was guilty of having neglected old and vulnerable patients and had failed to provide a suitable environment for their care.

The respondent was not present at the hearing of the charges and was not represented in her absence although it was adequately demonstrated that the formal notice of the hearing had been served. There having been no written admission, a number of witness had to be called to describe the circumstances referred to above. Having questioned the witnesses the Committee was satisfied that the charges were proved and constituted misconduct in a professional sense. Do you agree with those conclusions?

It was not possible to provide the Committee with any previous history concerning the respondent since she appeared to have been self-employed in that she was running her own business for not only the tenure of this nursing home but other nursing homes before it. She had not been the subject of any previous proven misconduct by any of the statutory bodies. The respondent had been told that the opportunity would exist for her to place evidence in mitigation before the Committee. She had not responded and the Committee was therefore placed in considerable difficulty in that they had neither seen her nor heard evidence from other people in support of her continued registration.

You are now to see yourselves as members of the Professional Conduct Committee and, given that the facts were proved and considered misconduct, decide which of the available three decisions you consider appropriate to the case. You might also consider what lessons emerge from the case and whether you would wish to make any recommendations to the authority with which the nursing home was registered in respect of its inspection arrangements.

CASE A9

An experienced midwife appeared before the Professional Conduct Committee of the UKCC alleged to be guilty of misconduct in a professional sense. The charges stated that she administered Monotard and Actrapid by injection to a diabetic patient without following the correct procedure and when those drugs had not been prescribed. The allegations were denied. The respondent was present and represented by a barrister so the evidence of the witnesses was thoroughly tested in cross-examination.

The patient was admitted to hospital for an elective Caesarian section operation. It was normal practice to admit such patients on the day prior to operation and to starve them from midnight. The patient was an established diabetic who had been taking insulin at home in the form of Monotard 40 units and Actrapid 16 units daily at 7.30 AM. Admission records were made by a student midwife and a junior doctor, both of whom noted in their records the patient's established insulin regime.

The operation was performed the next day. On that day a senior doctor prescribed 500 ml of 10% dextrose with potassium chloride and 10 units of Actrapid insulin each six hours. Later that day the dose of Actrapid in each 500 ml of 10% dextrose was reduced to 5 units. Both prescriptions were properly recorded in the prescription sheet for intravenous fluids and additivies.

The respondent was on night duty on the relevant ward for the night following the patient's operation. Another midwifery sister was in charge of the whole maternity unit for that night. On her round at 10 PM she discussed the patient's management with the respondent and enquired of her what treatment the patient was receiving and how often blood sugars should be done. She recalled asking the respondent whether she knew what the normal level was and receiving a negative answer. She told the respondent to contact the house officer. The same witness also recalled (1) asking the respondent if the patient was to recommence her insulin injections in the morning and the respondent saying that she was; and (2) visiting the ward later when the respondent told her that she had contacted the house officer and had been told the normal blood sugar reading using the Reflomat test.

This sister and other witnesses described the arrangements for prescribing and administering drugs in the hospital. There was a form headed 'Prescription Sheet' with a section for drugs to be given once only and another for continuing prescriptions. This document showed the local policy to be that drugs were to be administered only in accordance with prescriptions written on that prescription sheet. Records of drugs administered were kept on a 'Drug Recording Sheet', which contained two statements to the effect that those administering drugs should refer to the prescription sheet for the details of the dose and route of administration. In addition there was a further prescription sheet for 'Intravenous Fluids and Additives'. The procedure document for the health authority was widely available and a copy was in the drugs trolley.

At 7.30 AM on the morning after the operation, the respondent administered 40 units of Monotard and 16 units of Actrapid although this had not been prescribed by any doctor and there was no entry concerning it on the prescription sheet. She made a clear entry on the 'Drug Recording Sheet' that these drugs had been given. At the change of shift the day sister received the night report from the respondent and, at 7.50 AM, was told by the respondent that she had given the patient her 'Insulin dose of 40 units Monotard and 16 units Actrapid'. The day sister commented that the patient was not yet eating and was continuing to receive intravenous therapy of 'dextrose and potassium chloride and 5 units of Actrapid in each 500 ml'. The respondent said that she had followed the doses stated in the patient's notes. It was pointed out to her by the day sister that those entries in both the clinical and nursing notes were part of the admission history and not instructions or prescriptions for that insulin to be administered as an inpatient. Contrary to local policy, no other member of staff had been involved in checking or observing the administration of the drug.

The Council's solicitor called the patient and six other witnesses, all of whom were cross-examined by the barrister on behalf of the respondent and questioned by the Committee members. At the end of the 'Did It Happen' stage of the hearing the Committee found the allegations proved to the strict standard of proof required.

The respondent's barrister then argued that the Committee should not regard the facts proved as misconduct because (in her view) bad practices prevailed in the hospital, the drugs procedure was poor, the prescriptions were 'dismal' and the error was a 'one-off' in a long career. The Committee did, however, find the facts proved to constitute professional misconduct.

The Committee then received information about the respondent's previous history and the material that she wished to submit in mitigation. The midwifery manager for the health authority said that she had known the respondent for seven years, though not particularly well, having only recently stepped into a role that gave her closer contact. She said that the midwife had first been appointed as a special care sister because she had experience in that field and had obtained the Midwife Teachers Diploma. She moved to the main midwifery unit six months after appointment because she needed to do part-time night duty to fit in with her husband's studies. The witness confirmed that, during the respondent's employment she would have encountered diabetic patients on the maternity unit with reasonable frequency since they were cared for in the normal maternity wards. The witness summarised the respondent as being 'a pretty average midwife' and indicated that such criticism as there had been related not to her professional work but to her general attitude towards her work.

In mitigation from the respondent it emerged that, prior to undertaking a Midwife Teachers Diploma, she had been active in teaching student midwives and in planning and organising their courses. While working on night duty and seeking to organise her life to fit in with her husband's studies, the respondent had also been a mature student and had obtained a BA degree at polytechnic. She had continued her studies and obtained an MA and was now undertaking studies for a PhD. Although well qualified academically and continuing her advanced studies, the respondent indicated that she hoped and expected to use her nursing and midwifery qualifications again, though not necessarily in the clinical setting. Three letters of testimonial in support of the respondent were submitted.

Put yourself in the position of the members who served on the Professional Conduct Committee. You have before you a highly qualified professional nurse and midwife. You have proved her guilty of misconduct in a professional sense for a fairly basic error which she did not recognise to be such and which occurred when all the available information and a question raised by her superior should have helped her to avoid it. She is not in current nursing or midwifery practice but has declared to you her intention to use again the registration which she wishes to retain.

Consider also whether other people contributed to this occurrence and should be made the subject of criticism in the announcement of the decision and what lessons emerge from this case that might be applied in your own work setting. Indeed, ask yourself 'Could this happen where I work?' and 'What do I need to do to avoid it happening?'

CASE A10

A 43-year-old health visitor (RGN/RHV) appeared unrepresented before the Professional Conduct Committee facing 17 charges alleging misconduct. Two charges alleged failure to keep a record of official mileage for which reimbursement was claimed, four alleged failure to keep health visiting records in respect of visits, two alleged failure to record the results of hearing tests, two alleged failure to record the results of developmental screening, three alleged failure to record on primary record cards the results of phenylketonuria tests, two alleged failure to forward immunisation consent forms to the relevant sections and the final two alleged failure to forward data sheets to the Pre-School Health Section.

The respondent admitted the facts but required the evidence to be heard before the Committee adjudicated upon the matter of misconduct.

The evidence revealed that, three years after she had taken up the health visitor post in question (having moved from a similar post with the adjacent health authority) the respondent was on holiday. At this stage, there having been some difficulty with a disparity between caseloads, a count was undertaken with a view to reallocation. As the respondent was on leave and had not completed her part of the count the nursing officer obtained access to her records. She discovered discrepancies. Together with a colleague, she then carried out a detailed investigation. This revealed considerable problems in respect of the records. Some had no entries. Some development test reports had not been entered on the records. Some vaccination and immunisation consent forms had not been passed on. When the respondent's diary was checked it was noted that she had not kept any record of the mileage for which she had sought reimbursement. When these matters were put to her by her manager she could give no explanation.

In her evidence to the Committee the nursing officer (to whom the respondent had been responsible) defined the basic duties of the health visitor as 'To home visit mothers and babies, antenatally and up to five years old, and then school nursing and teenagers if necessary; to perform routine development screening, and offer advice and support to the care of mothers and young babies.' She told the committee that four health visitors worked in her area, with average caseloads of 400 children 0–5. The witness also told the committee that it was local policy that diaries be used to record visits, trips, lectures given and mileage travelled. Other policies related to developmental assessments on a 9–18–36-month plan, hearing tests to be performed between seven and nine months, and the recording of PKU test results. In respect of immunisation an offer was made to all parents, and where they consented the consent form was sent to the Vaccination and Immunisation Department who sent an appointment for the child to be taken to the appropriate clinic.

It was against her statement of the role and the local policies that the nursing officer had found the respondent wanting, in that there were primary record cards of some two-year-old children with no entries, some three-year-old children with no entries after 9 months, cards with no PKU results recorded or attached or with no hearing test and/or developmental test entries made. A quantity of PKU reports were found in a drawer. It should be noted, however, that the same witness had called in the cards annually for a check on the distribution of work, and had not previously observed the deficiencies since she simply did a count of the cards, and not an examination of even a sample of them.

In response to the questions from the Committee the witness said that the HV service was organised on a GP attachment basis where a patient moved into a HV's area but retained her GP in another area by arrangement, and that the annual review was of workload (including time spent at antenatal classes, parentcraft classes, clinics, GP work, and health education) and not just caseload. It also became clear that health visitors completed a monthly return as to how many hearing tests they had done in the period, but this (she said) did not contain names and did not serve as a check on individual HV record cards.

Pressed by a member of the Committee about her responsibility to monitor the work of her staff and her manner of doing it, the witness said that health visitors were highly trained practitioners, so she would not do planned monitoring visits, but if there was ever a complaint she would follow it up and then perhaps look at a random sample of record cards. Since she had received no complaint about the respondent she had done no such sampling. The witness also confirmed that in the light of this case the whole system of monitoring, management and induction had changed, and that although the plan was to undertake formal appraisal of health visitors annually this had never happened with this employee in her four years with that authority.

In her own evidence the respondent drew attention to the fact that the nursing officer's evidence had failed to indicate that it was required that each HV keep a birth book with details of each child born in or moving into the area, that it also should be checked by nurse managers, and that in that book there were columns for recording PKU results, hearing and developmental test results, and the move to school or out of the area. Her records in that respect were complete. She challenged the nursing officer's statement about the monthly return regarding hearing tests, stating that there were individual sheets attached to the monthly return, and that these indicated whether it was a first or second test, the result, and whether the case was being referred on to the community physician. She similarly and quite effectively challenged some other aspects of the nursing officer's evidence.

The respondent confirmed that she had not maintained the records referred to in the charges, but that she was contesting that she was guilty of misconduct on certain of the charges since she had made records of those matters in other documents which the health authority also required her to keep. It was clear that she could speak in a detailed manner about the children and families which could only have been the result of frequent visits and great interest in them.

In spite of the respondent's submission, the Committee considered the facts in respect of all charges to be misconduct. The hearing moved to the stage where evidence in mitigation or aggravation is heard. The director of nursing services gave details of the respondent's record in general nursing, industrial nursing and health visiting prior to taking the post in which the charges arose. Her career appeared to have been exemplary. The reference from her previous HV post referred to some tension with colleagues, but also to her strength as a leader and her leadership qualities. This witness said that she had met the respondent on a few occasions only, but had found her intelligent and stimulating. She referred to her innovative ideas and approach, and told the committee of a course she had run for her colleagues to demonstrate counselling techniques which was 'excellent and received the highest praise from all who attended'. She went on to say that when she interviewed the respondent about the gaps in her records she failed to grasp the enormity of her failure or to provide an explanation, so she dismissed her from employment.

Pressed by the Committee, the same witness agreed that one of her interviews had been at the request of the respondent who had brought with her a critical analysis of herself which exposed her problem regarding paperwork and documentation, and stated that as a result she instructed the nursing officer to 'chase her up for her monthly statistics'.

In her own address in mitigation the respondent spoke of the practical problems she had overcome as a single parent to train as a health visitor, but that she bore those burdens to take up the career of her choice. She accepted responsibility for her failures, but felt that the response to them had been excessive since she had worked satisfactorily as a HV in other places. She had on taking up her post, found that relationships between the various professionals involved (two GP practices operating from the same base) were 'stormy' and stated that she had tried to be a mediator. Although there was a part-time clerk to do some clerical work for the HVs, because the previous staff had not used her she (being conscientious) had filled her time with other health centre work which she then could not shed. In any case, her skills did not include shorthand or audio typing. Attempts to get the nursing officer to come to talk about these problems had failed. She said that the general attitude of the managers was that 'If you are finding it difficult you are not good enough for the job'. She gave details of a number of innovations which had been a feature of her practice, and which were clearly impressive.

A clinical psychologist who attended as a friend of the respondent confirmed the problems of the health centre and the many difficulties arising from staff attitudes and staff changes and spoke of the high level of concern and high standard of care the respondent provided for her clients. Numerous testimonials were also submitted.

The Committee members felt that they had before them a committed, articulate, innovative health visitor, but one who also needed the sort of manager who would help keep her feet on the ground and ensure that basic tasks were done before advancing into new territory, while still encouraging innovation.

You know that the facts are admitted and are seen as misconduct. What will you now do by way of passing judgment?

CASE A11

A 35-year-old registered mental nurse appeared before the Professional Conduct Committee as a result of an incident alleged to have occurred in the Psycho-Geriatric Assessment Ward of which she was the sister.

The Committee noted that her managers were convinced that she had struck an elderly incontinent patient on the face with a 'Comfipad' intended to be used when she was being dressed. The respondent's professional managers dismissed her from employment but did not report her to the statutory bodies (to enable the question of whether she should lose or retain her registration status to be considered) until the sister won an appeal against dismissal. What is your view of this?

The incident was alleged to have occurred at 7.30 AM. The ward consisted of two dormitories (one for the 15 more dependent patients and the other for the less dependent), with offices, kitchen, linen cupboards, etc. between the dormitories. There was agreement between all witnesses that the day shift commenced when they came on at 7.00 AM, received the report and then discussed the work and patients over a drink. This brought the time to approximately 7.25 AM.

The nursing was undertaken on a strict task allocation basis, the first task for all staff being to get all patients up and dressed for breakfast which was served at a strict 8.00 AM. This being the case, work tended to be rushed during the 35–40 minute period available.

On this morning, into the dormitory for the more dependent patients went the sister (the respondent in this case), an enrolled nurse, a student nurse and a nursing assistant. The sister instructed her staff which patient each of them should get up and dress first, herself taking the patient who was alleged to have been struck, having been told by the enrolled nurse that she had struggled alone with this patient for the previous three mornings while the sister had been off and did not wish to do so again. The practice on the ward was that the nurses worked alone in the belief that this achieved results more quickly.

It emerged that although the dormitory had curtain rails and curtains intended to provide privacy for patients they were useless since the dormitory was used for more beds than planned so the curtain rails were fixed either at the centre of the bedhead or behind the wardrobes adjacent to the beds. However, because there were curtains the dormitory had no screens!

The situation therefore, was of nurses simultaneously getting patients undressed, out of bed, sat upon commodes, and eventually dressed with no privacy. Given the type of patients accommodated in this dormitory, the noise level was considerable, but it was supplemented by the radio. Over all of this the nurses shared shouted conversation aimed at bringing the sister up-to-date with information concerning the patients during her days off.

What is your view of this scenario and those responsible for it?

Picture the scene. The sister is working half way along one side of the dormitory. She has got her patient out of bed and that patient is now sitting partly clothed on a commode by the side of her bed, facing towards her wardrobe which is adjacent to the head of the bed. The sister is between the patient (facing her) and the wardrobe. The patient is described as suffering from senile dementia, as having a right hemiplegia, and as being heavy.

The student nurse is similarly placed with a patient on a commode adjacent to her bed on the same side of the ward and approximately 20 feet away. The other two staff have reached an exactly similar stage with their respective patients on the other side of the dormitory. They are each about 15 feet away from the sister's patient in diagonal directions. There is no obstruction to the view of any of the nursing staff, no curtains or screens being in use.

The item of furniture next to each patient's bed was a narrow wardrobe with a lower level locker section. The ward routine was that at the end of a day the staff made up a bundle of clothes ready for the patient the next morning, placing it with a 'Comfipad' on the locker top.

The student and the assistant gave evidence to the effect that, after speaking to the patient loudly and in a cross manner the sister hit her across the face with the pad. The student said it was folded fairly tight with the plastic surface outwards at the time of contact. The assistant described it as held in one hand and more than half opened, and also gave evidence of loud, cross words. The enrolled nurse said she heard no loud or cross words above the normal noise level of the ward. She described the sister as holding the patient with one hand on her shoulder and reaching behind her to take the folded 'Comfipad' from the locker with her right hand, shaking it vigorously, and then bringing it across the front of the patient to place it in readiness on the bed.

The sister said that whereas the patient could sit safely on a chair with a slight backward tilt, she tipped forward on a commode unless held by one shoulder, and at some stages of the proceedings with a knee held against her legs. She denied any cross words, but said it was necessary to speak to the patient loudly as she was quite deaf. Her description of the movement of the 'Comfipad' was the same as that of the enrolled nurse, and she denied any contact with the patient as she brought the pad across.

The two who believed that they had seen the patient struck said or did nothing. Later in the day, when placing the patient in the bath together, they called the staff nurse (then in charge) to examine a sore area on the patient's leg which required dressing. While she was with them they told her what they believed they had heard and seen. She reported it to her managers with the consequence stated above.

Evidence at the Committee is given under oath and must be direct evidence only – not hearsay. The standard of proof required before finding an alleged incident proved is that the Committee members must be satisfied so that they are sure.

In this case would you, given this evidence, consider that the allegations were proved to the required standard? If yes, would you consider those matters to be misconduct in a professional sense? If yes to that, what would be your judgment on this ward sister?

Whatever your answers to those questions you can also make representations to the health authority in the person of its chairman and/or its professional managers by sending a verbatim transcript of the hearing and drawing attention to the matters that have caused you concern. Do you want to do that? What concerns would you express?

CASE A12

Three experienced nurses (one enrolled nurse, one ward sister and one nursing officer) from a general hospital ward were the subject of a joint hearing before the Professional Conduct Committee which stretched over two long days. All denied the allegations made against them.

The enrolled nurse was alleged to have struck one elderly patient, to have treated another patient in a rough and unkind manner, and to have made derogatory remarks of a sectarian nature to a teenage patient who was hospitalized far from home.

The ward sister was alleged to have failed properly to investigate two of those matters which had been the subject of complaints made to her by the teenage patient's mother and a student nurse respectively.

The nursing officer was alleged to have failed properly to investigate the alleged rough and unkind treatment, and in effect to have colluded with the ward sister in a cover-up when that allegation was relentlessly pursued by the concerned student nurse.

The cases began to emerge for consideration only when that student nurse wrote to the statutory nursing bodies, her local representations seeking investigation of and action concerning the enrolled nurse's alleged reprehensible conduct having seemingly failed. By this time a staff nurse in her first post (with the same employment authority), she wrote to the National Board to allege misconduct against the above mentioned three practitioners, and also a senior nursing officer. The latter's case was not forwarded for hearing by the Investigating Committee, but she did find herself called in evidence.

When the Council's solicitor began to investigate the matters alleged, two more former student nurses (by then staff nurses) volunteered evidence of the 'striking' incident, as did the young patient. The two nurses and another colleague provided evidence about the atmosphere on the ward.

The witness who originated the allegations told the Committee how she had seen the enrolled nurse repeatedly poke an elderly patient and physically throw her into a chair. She said she was taken aback as she had never seen anything like it before. She was troubled by what she had seen, but found it difficult to raise the matter with the sister, as the two sisters and enrolled nurse of that ward seemed to constitute an inner circle from which all other staff were excluded. After three weeks of agonising (overlapping with studying for finals) she felt she could keep silence no longer, told the enrolled nurse she intended to complain to the sister about what she had observed, and did exactly that. She said that the sister told her she would investigate the matter and come back to her.

The combination of moving from the ward, studying for final examinations, eventually passing and becoming a staff nurse pushed the matter to the back of her mind until she overheard the conversation of some student nurses (who had recently passed through the ward in question) which led her to believe that comparable incidents were still occurring. As a result she wrote to the sister, reminded her of the incident she had reported and the date, reminded her of the undertaking to investigate and report, and courteously asked what transpired.

She did not receive a reply from the sister or the nursing officer, but from the senior nursing officer. That letter said that the matter had been investigated and resolved, but gave no information. The young staff nurse wrote back to express surprise since she was the complainant and she had not been asked for a statement, and again courteously asked the nature of the investigation. The response she received again provided no information, but suggested she make an appointment to see the senior nursing officer. This she did, and when she went to that appointment after night duty she was faced by the senior nursing officer and the nursing officer. She received no answers to her questions, but felt she was faced with pressure to accept that the complaint had been investigated and resolved, and to pursue the matter no further. It was following that interview that she wrote to the Board to allege misconduct.

Corroborative evidence about the atmosphere on the ward came from the other student nurses. One said 'I felt the sisters and enrolled nurse were like a little unit on their own and the rest of us were outsiders'. Two of those witnesses also provided evidence of the alleged striking incident. The young patient and her mother provided evidence of the derogatory sectarian remarks, which in turn had led to a second complaint to the sister which it had been alleged had not been investigated.

In respect of the nursing officer, it was alleged that she had accepted the sister's conviction that the roughness/unkindness had not happened, finding this possible because she also had known the enrolled nurse for some years. It emerged in evidence that two undated documents which purported to indicate that an investigation had taken place subsequently appeared in the enrolled nurse's file, but the fact remained that the complainant had not been asked for a statement.

After nearly two days of evidence for and against the allegations the Committee found all of them proved to their satisfaction. There seemed to be absolutely no reason why the witnesses should go to such lengths and personal inconvenience to support fabricated stories. Having found the allegations proved the Committee considered them all to be misconduct in a professional sense.

At the mitigation/aggravation stage of the hearing the Committee learnt that, once the original allegation letter to the Board had been copied by the complainant to the director of nursing services, earnest efforts had been taken to investigate and take action in respect of the three respondents.

None of the three had been dismissed from employment, but the management had taken steps in respect of each of them which were brought to the attention of the Committee. In respect of the enrolled nurse, the employers seemingly recognised that she had become institutionalised and her judgment impaired through working for so long in one specific ward, and had arranged a refresher course following which she was relocated to another ward. Evidence was received that her performance was being closely monitored in that work situation, and that she was performing well. Excellent references were received about her performance in general, and it was believed that she was normally regarded as a kind person.

In respect of the ward sister, it was brought to the attention of the Committee that her employers had arranged for her to undertake a development programme following which she had returned to her ward where it was believed she now recognised her failure to handle properly the matters which were the substance of the charges, and had earned the confidence of her director of nursing services.

In respect of the nursing officer, the managers, recognising that she had been thrust into a nursing officer role without preparation and at a time when no senior nursing officer was in post, had provided her with management training, enabled her to attend a variety of seminars and study days, and actively involved her in drawing up policies in the areas in which they believed she had demonstrated a deficiency. Again it was brought to the attention of the Committee through references that she was tackling her post with enthusiasm, and had demonstrated a new initiative in embarking on part-time studies for a degree.

The members of the Committee obviously had to feel concern about each of the three practitioners whom they had found guilty as alleged, and guilty of misconduct in a professional sense. The enrolled nurse they saw as having abrogated her responsibility of care, in that she handled patients in a manner alien to the standard of practice expected of a qualified nurse. In addition, she had failed to satisfy the requirement of the Code of Professional Conduct that she accord respect due to the customs, values and spiritual beliefs of a patient. In respect of the ward sister, they saw her as having on two occasions, demonstrated a failure to take seriously and investigate properly complaints made to her, the substance of which were very serious. She had failed to satisfy a prime responsibility to ensure that the standards of practice on her ward were maintained to a high level, and failed to monitor what went on in the ward. The members were in no doubt that the proper investigation of complaints is a component of fulfilling the responsibilities of a ward sister, and any views held by the person about the competence and standards of a member of staff should not influence her when complaints are brought. In respect of the nursing officer, the members deplored the fact that she had been thrust into the nursing officer role without appropriate training or induction, and without appropriate support, and believed that her employers had placed her in an impossible position. Although she had responded extremely unwisely to a situation which had developed, it was felt that she had been placed by her employers in an extremely difficult position.

See yourself as a member of the Professional Conduct Committee. You have before you three persons who have, in their respective ways, failed to behave appropriately, and you have found the allegations against them (which they denied) to be proved and have regarded them as misconduct. You have also heard something of the management context within which they offended, and the things said in mitigation. Now you must decide whether, in respect of each of them, you would postpone your judgment on the matter for a stated period and set any criteria to be satisfied for a resumed hearing, or remove from the register or take no action apart from giving advice on standards of conduct.

In addition to that, ask yourself whether this could happen in the place in which you work or for which you have a managerial responsibility, and use it as a stimulus to examine your own practice.

CASE A13

The Professional Conduct Committee of the United Kingdom Central Council considered the case of a 31-year-old registered nurse and registered midwife who was the subject of a charge of professional misconduct, and who therefore stood at risk of losing her right to practise.

The incident that led to the particular charge occurred some months earlier, at night, in a special care baby unit located within a labour ward suite. The unit had originally been designed to accommodate 13 babies, but for some time had been used for 18. One consequence of this was that, with not only the required number of cots, but also incubators, ventilators, infusion and monitoring equipment, etc., the unit was grossly overcrowded and presented the staff with severe problems.

On the night in question there were 18 babies in the unit, of whom two were being supported by ventilators, six were in incubators, and six having intravenous infusions. The number of staff on duty was five, of which four were described as midwives and the other as an enrolled nurse. There was no additional cover for mealtimes.

The charge alleging misconduct stated that the respondent had incorrectly administered a low birth weight infant feed to a baby through an intravenous line. This unfortunate error had tragic consequences.

The registered nurse/midwife admitted the facts of the charge, but (through the barrister representing her) indicated her intention to contest that, in the particular circumstances of the case, her unfortunate mistake amounted to professional misconduct.

The Committee therefore received detailed information concerning the operation of the unit in question, and heard evidence from expert witnesses in respect of the management of such units and their staffing needs.

The expert evidence indicated that, even in a unit which was well designed and laid out so as to facilitate observation and care, 18 babies of this degree of dependence would require a staff of not less than seven at any given time. Those staff would need to be deployed so as to maintain continuity of observation and care, which would necessitate the allocation of several babies to each member of the trained staff. When shown photographs of the unit in question the expert witnesses expressed the view that it was grossly overcrowded in a way which would render good care and observation more difficult, require more staff to achieve it, and make patient allocation even more important.

The Committee members were informed that, on the night in question, one of the patients was a baby who, at his birth 28 days earlier, had weighed 2 lb. He had been making reasonable progress, but was still having occasional apnoea attacks. He was in an incubator, on constant oxygen, had an intravenous infusion into a scalp vein, a naso-gastric tube and a cardiac monitor. At 10.00 PM one member of staff, while giving care and taking observations, noticed that the intravenous infusion had 'tissued'. A doctor was called, and inserted a new needle to recommence the infusion. However, because the lumen of the new vessel was smaller he did not think it able to accommodate all the fluids being administered. The infusion had been used to administer Parenterovite and Interlipid. The doctor stopped the Interlipid, and used a small syringe to close the inlet port at the multiple connector in the infusion line. The Interlipid had been in the process of administration from a syringe within a pump placed on top of the incubator.

Also on top of the incubator, in another syringe of the same size, and in a similar syringe pump, was the low birth weight infant feed, placed ready for use by another member of the staff. Neither syringe was labelled, and this was in accordance with the normal practice in the unit; a practice certainly known to its senior manager. The contents of both syringes were white liquids.

The regime in the unit was such that particular members of staff were not allocated to care for specific babies. Instead the observation and care of a particular baby became the responsibility of whoever happened to be available at the time. For the patient in question, half-hourly observations over a two-hour period were performed by four different members of staff. It was also learned that the permanent core staff in the unit were very few, all midwives in the department being allocated as circumstances demanded and allowed. The unit had been meant to have one more midwife on the night in question, but she was reallocated because the labour ward was busy.

This, then, was the setting within which, at 11.00 PM one night, the respondent in this case unfortunately connected the infant feed to the intravenous line rather than the nasogastric tube, and in which three of her colleagues who undertook observations at the next three half-hourly intervals, and a doctor who attended when the apnoea attacks became more frequent, failed to recognise the error, because of the similarity of the liquids.

In the view of the expert witnesses and the Committee the unit was grossly overcrowded, critically understaffed, devoid of a reasonable regime for managing and delivering care, and desperately in need of a staffing plan which prevented the babies being placed at risk by demands elsewhere in the department. In short, it was a place with an accident waiting to happen.

You might care to consider how (had you been a member of the Professional Conduct Committee) you would have voted in response to the submission that, given the appalling circumstances of this case, the admitted factors should not be regarded as professional misconduct.

Whether or not you engage in that exercise, surely you must consider whether an incident like this could happen where you work or in a place for which you have management responsibility.

CASE A14

Two registered general nurses, each with over 25 years experience, faced a joint hearing before the Professional Conduct Committee. The circumstances that led them to be there had been that, some weeks before, while on duty at night in a very busy medical unit of a large general hospital, they had admitted a seriously ill young woman.

The woman had been suffering from postnatal depression which had culminated in her ingesting a large overdose of paracetamol tablets. On her admission to a ward within the medical unit it was believed that she had ingested the tablets at least 12 hours earlier. The sister (who had responsibility for the four wards in the medical unit at night) and the staff nurse (whose only assistance was from one nursing auxiliary) expressed concern to the doctor involved about the admission of the patient to the ward in question. First, they expressed the view that her admission would mean that their inability to properly care for the 28 patients they had would be made even greater. Second, they pointed out that in the nearby intensive care unit there was room, staff, equipment and expertise to better cope with such an emergency situation. The doctor rejected their views, said that the patient must stay there and that treatment by an intravenous infusion of Parvolex must be commenced immediately. While the doctor was writing a prescription, the sister and staff nurse went to the drug cupboard and produced all that they had of the drug being prescribed. The doctor meanwhile wrote a proper prescription for 9000 mg by intravenous infusion. When the nurses came from the cupboard with all the stock they had (which would have been adequate) the doctor said that it was 'not enough to treat a mouse', and rushed out of the ward door to use his emergency key to open the pharmacy. He returned carrying a large quantity of packets of the drug. He then opened one of the cartons and lifted up an ampoule on which he saw in bold print '200 mg'; he said that this meant that they needed to give 45 of these 10 ml ampoules. The nurses were surprised at this, since it seemed such a large volume but went ahead with their preparations, and, over a period of time, added the Parvolex from the ampoules to the infusion which had been established.

Most of the Parvolex had been infused before the patient began to demonstrate other serious symptoms, which led to the remainder not being given and to the patient then being moved to the intensive care unit where she died during the next 24 hours. Subsequent to her developing the further symptoms it was realised in discussion that she had been given a substantial overdose.

A complaint about the night sister and the staff nurse was brought. The Investigating Committee considered it and had before them statements from the two nurses in which they admitted frankly that it had all happened as described. The two cases were forwarded for hearing before the Professional Conduct Committee. Had you been the Investigating Committee would you have made the same decision?

At the joint hearing the two nurses, through their legal representatives, admitted the allegations in the charges as to fact, but indicated they wished to challenge the suggestion that it constituted misconduct. The representatives then presented cogent argument, illustrated by a number of important points. These included:

(1) the unreasonable pressure of the work in the medical unit at the time in question;
(2) the fact that such pressure had been continuous for a substantial period of time – a letter sent by them to the director of nursing services (together with a further document to which reference is made below) some eight months earlier together with a totally unsympathetic and unhelpful reply was produced in evidence;

(3) the fact that the doctor had also made a mistake and compounded it by his actions (and he was not the subject of a complaint to his regulating body);

(4) the fact that, at the inquest, the coroner also misread the ampoules and cartons to indicate 200 mg per ampoule when it was in fact 200 mg per ml in each 10 ml ampoule;

(5) the fact that in consequence of this case and several like it, the manufacturers had completely changed the labelling of both ampoules and cartons (examples of both were produced to the Committee).

The document which had been sent by the two nurses to the director of nursing services was of particular significance, in that they had taken a great deal of their personal time and applied their considerable experience to prepare a brilliant document which was based on their detailed assessment of the 130 patients in the unit on a particular (but typical) day. This clearly showed how great was the gap between needs and resources.

See yourself as the Professional Conduct Committee. How would you have answered the question 'Is this misconduct?' If you say 'yes' you should have a view as to the subsequent judgment you would then pass on two nurses whose careers to that time had been exemplary, and who had tried to fulfil their responsibilities under the Code of Conduct.

CASE A15

A registered general nurse who was a very experienced operating theatre sister came before the Professional Conduct Committee of the UKCC to answer an allegation arising out of an incident in the course of her work.

The circumstances of the case were that, in an operating theatre for which she had responsibility and where she had been a scrub/instrument nurse for a sequence of cases, there had been a long and busy day. The final case on the list involving an abdominal operation for an elderly gentleman was completed only at the very end of the day shift, and the sister cleared the instruments away and put them into the automatic washer within the theatre suite, told the two members of the night staff who came on duty that this had been done, and requested that they remove them later. The evidence was that the two nurses on night duty had subsequently removed the set of instruments from the washer and laid them out on a tray to check, at which stage they found that one Dunhill forceps was missing from the set. They stated that they boldly labelled the tray to this effect in the event that they did not see the sister (the respondent nurse in the case) personally in the morning.

As it transpired they did see her and told her that the set was one instrument short and that they had therefore kept the incomplete set together on a tray which was boldly labelled to this effect, and which they now drew to her attention. It was said in evidence that the sister's reaction was that it could not be as they described, since she was always meticulous about her instrument checks. Having drawn attention to the matter and completed their shift of duty, the night nurses left.

The regulations covering that theatre suite required that, should it be necessary to draw an instrument from the reserve stocks to make up a set, this should only be done by calling in the nursing officer responsible for that set of theatres, or the sister/charge nurse acting up in her absence. This did not happen in this case, since the evidence showed that the sister had subsequently found the set was indeed deficient through the absence of the Dunhill forceps, and drew a replacement from the reserves without the involvement of any other person, and without informing either any member of the surgical team involved or her superiors.

Three weeks later the patient died from something unrelated to the surgery which he had undergone, but in circumstances requiring a post-mortem examination. In the course of the post-mortem a Dunhill forceps was found in the patient's abdominal cavity, as a result of which some enquiries ensued about the circumstances of the operation. The information set out above in respect of the missing instrument and the replacement from the reserve stock then emerged.

Faced with this situation the decision of the employing authority had been to dismiss the theatre sister from employment and to report the matter to the statutory bodies as a result of which the Professional Conduct Committee hearing was taking place. The allegation (which was to the effect that the sister had failed in her responsibility when it was reported to her that an instrument was missing, and acted to conceal the incident) was denied, but was proved on the evidence. It was also argued by the respondent and her representative that the Committee should not deem that which they had found proved to be misconduct in a professional sense.

Consider how you would have responded had you had to determine whether these now proven facts constituted misconduct in a professional sense. Consider also your reasons for whichever decision you make.

In the event the Committee determined that it did regard those facts as misconduct, so the case progressed to the stage at which evidence in mitigation or aggravation is heard. It emerged that the respondent had worked in theatre nursing continuously since her registration some 12 years earlier, had been employed as a theatre sister in a number of famous hospitals in this country and overseas, and was if anything regarded by her last employers as having been almost obsessional about her instrument checking to the neglect of some of her other responsibilities as a sister. It also emerged that the practice in the theatre suite in question was that, whilst the swabs were subject to a check involving several persons, responsibility for the instruments had rested with the instrument nurse alone, though the latter practice had been changed in the light of the case.

It also emerged that, very soon after dismissal from her employment the respondent had obtained a post as a theatre sister in a private hospital some 50 miles away. It appears that they were so delighted when approached by a very experienced theatre nurse that they had not taken up a reference from her previous employer. Although she had come to the hearing with an excellent open reference concerning her competence as a theatre nurse from her new employers, it also became clear in questioning that the reference was written without knowledge of the incident which led the respondent to be before the Committee.

Now place yourself in the role of a Professional Conduct Committee member again. What decision will you make?

CASE A16

A newly qualified registered sick children's nurse, aged 21 years, came before the Professional Conduct Committee as a result of incidents occurring in the paediatric ward where she was employed as a staff nurse on night duty.

On completing her training successfully she found that there were no staff nurse posts available in the area she knew, so she had no alternative but to study national advertisements. She made application to an authority several hundred miles from her familiar setting, and travelled to take up her post.

Although taking up a post in her own paediatric speciality she was in all other respects a stranger in a setting in which staff turnover was very limited. She had an induction programme of three days duration, following which she was placed in charge of a paediatric ward on night duty. The incident which led to her dismissal and to her subsequent appearance before the committee occurred only a few weeks later.

On the night in question she was in charge of a busy 25-bed ward with a number of very ill children (for example, three in cubicles had meningitis), with support staff of one pupil nurse and one auxiliary, and with knowledge of the fact that the night sister covering her ward was not a specialist paediatric nurse.

At approximately midnight she became concerned about the condition of a particular baby and decided that some suction was indicated. She took the baby to the treatment room, only to find that the fitted suction equipment was not operating. Fearing that the baby was deteriorating, she carried him quickly to another location where there was some portable suction equipment and again attempted to pass a tube. She had difficulty and believed this might be the result of congestion in the nasal and upper respiratory passages. She decided (a) to administer 2 drops of Otrivine to each nostril (knowing that it was not prescribed), (b) to call the doctor, and (c) to call the cardiac arrest team, which she did in that order. She also repeated her attempted suction, this time successfully.

When others arrived they determined that there had not been an arrest, and that the baby was now satisfactory. The doctor for the paediatric unit was not told by the staff nurse that she had given Otrivine drops, but as it happened wrote a prescription for such.

The staff nurse did not give the first prescribed dose but signed as having done so because she had given them prior to the prescription. This troubled the pupil nurse who subsequently mentioned it to a senior person, and an investigation ensued. In the course of that investigation it was noted that a few nights before, while not having the official authority to do so, the staff nurse had responded to pressure from a junior doctor to give some intravenous additives for her, and had quite clearly recorded that she had done so.

She was therefore charged with misconduct for giving an unprescribed drug, for not reporting that she had done so, for not giving the first prescribed dose, and her part in the matter of the IV additive. She had been dismissed by her employers.

The respondent did not deny the allegations, and was willing to accept that they could be regarded as misconduct, but told the Committee that on the night in question she genuinely thought that the baby was going to die and that she panicked, her experience of managing a crisis of this nature being none.

The committee received good references from her training school, and a report from the Nurses Welfare Service about her difficult family background and early departure from home. It also noted that she had not wasted her time since dismissal and while waiting for the hearing, but had taken up social work training at a polytechnic, whence came good reports and references. She had helped fund her course through part time auxiliary/assistant work in both health and social work settings.

The facts are admitted. Would you regard those facts as misconduct? If so what judgment will you pass on this young woman who has made it clear that, though preparing for a social work qualification, she wishes to retain her nurse status and possibly work at some future stage in a role that bridges both spheres.

CASE A17

A 50-year-old registered mental nurse appeared before the Committee to answer two charges arising out of matters relating to her work. She had been employed at a day centre which was a joint health and social services venture staffed by a full-time specialist social worker, two full-time nurses (one a charge nurse and the other being the respondent employed in a deputy charge nurse capacity), and several community service volunteers. In addition to their work in the centre the two registered nurses were also responsible for some home visits in the locality, particularly in respect of patients who attended the day centre.

One such patient around whom the charges revolved was an elderly lady who had become incapable of managing her own affairs and was the subject of a Court of Protection Order. She attended the centre and was also visited by the staff at home, and it therefore became well known to them (as to the specialist social worker on the team) that the patient (who lived alone) was having to move from a large family house into a much smaller dwelling. As a result of this it was going to be necessary for her to dispose of a considerable amount of furniture, having first decided what items she would retain for her smaller accommodation. Arrangements for an auction of the spare furniture were in the hands of a solicitor who was an agent for the Court of Protection.

It was alleged that the respondent nurse in this case identified some items of furniture which she would like to have for herself, and engaged in some form of barter both in face to face meetings with the patient and in telephone conversations. It was also alleged that, the day before the patient was to move to her smaller dwelling, the respondent made urgent arrangements for her husband to remove a number of items of furniture and instructed a young man who was one of the community service volunteers to accompany her husband with his van to the house, ensure that he was given directions and assist with the removal of the furniture. It was further alleged that the community service volunteer was given £100 in cash to give to the patient in exchange for the furniture, he also being required to indicate that more would follow later. He was subsequently given another sum of between £35 and £40 to pass on to the patient. Further to that, it was alleged that, when some time later, the story about the 'exchange' of a number of items of furniture (including a dining table and eight chairs, a chest of drawers and a plant stand) became known to the director of nursing services on receipt of a letter from the social worker, and when he in turn arranged to take the matter up with the respondent, the respondent sought to persuade the community service volunteer to state a false story in order to clear her.

It is important to note that the community service volunteer was a young man who had moved very far from his home in the North East of England because of difficulty in obtaining employment, that the event involving the exchange of furniture for money happened very early in his time at the centre, and that though recruited through social services he spent much of his time working at the centre with the nurses or going with them on visits where his assistance was required. With no previous knowledge of the world of work he had deemed it logical to do as the respondent instructed him in respect of the removal of the furniture, but he absolutely refused to be party to the fabrication of an untrue story, the essence of which was that he tell the director of nursing services that the furniture had really been for him to transfer to his parents who were existing in deprived conditions with very little furniture, and that the money was a loan to him from the respondent to pay for it.

The allegations were strongly denied by the respondent through her representative, but on the evidence of the community service volunteer and of the director of nursing services were found proved. The evidence of the latter was that of an interview with the respondent in which she had made it clear that she knew the patient's affairs were under the control of the Court of Protection and that this meant she was incapable of managing her own affairs and particularly her financial affairs. He indicated that he had elicited that she had known it was wrong to deal directly with the patient, and that she had made no attempt to deal through the solicitor.

The evidence of the community service volunteer was that the furniture was not his, had not been wanted by him, and that the money which exchanged hands was not money borrowed by him from the respondent in order to buy the furniture. He said that the respondent had raised the question of the furniture with the patient when he was present on a community visit, that the patient had said the furniture had to go to the sale rooms, and that though more substantial figures were at first mentioned the respondent had persuaded the patient to drop the price for all the items of furniture in which she was showing an interest to about £140.

The allegations having been found proved on the basis of the evidence and in spite of the respondent's denial, the Committee was addressed by the respondent's representative to the effect that these matters should not be regarded as misconduct. However, recognising the Code of Professional Conduct as the backcloth against which allegations of misconduct are judged, the Committee deemed those matters which they had proved to be clearly contrary to the introductory paragraph to the Code, and in particular to clauses 1 and 8, the latter of which states that each nurse (etc.) shall:

Avoid any abuse of the privileged relationship which exists with patients/ clients and of the privileged access allowed to their property, residence or workplace.

Consider first whether you would have regarded these proven offences as misconduct in a professional sense. Then accepting that misconduct was proved, consider what judgment (had you been a member of the Committee) you would then have made.

CASE A18

A 38-year-old registered general nurse and registered midwife appeared before the Professional Conduct Committee as a result of incidents arising from her employment as a practice nurse with a two partner practice.

The charges were to the effect that she stole two prescription forms from the practice, that she used these forms to attempt to obtain a quantity of medicines from a retail chemist and that she stole a sum of £445 from the practice.

The respondent did not attend the hearing and had not admitted the charges in writing subsequent to the formal notice calling the hearing. The evidence to support the charges was that of a police officer who was one of two called in to investigate as a result of a complaint from one of the doctors. This police officer had also been party to the arrest and interview of the respondent.

In respect of the money taken from the practice's business account, the evidence was that the respondent had paid into her personal account on the same day two cheques from the same account. One cheque, legitimately received and properly signed, was for her salary. The second, though dated the same day, was removed from a much lower place in the cheque book and the stub was not completed. The writing was not that of any of the authorised signatories. In the course of the interview the respondent denied all knowledge of that second cheque, even though her name was written on the back of the cheque and it featured with the legitimate cheque on the same paying-in slip.

In respect of the prescription forms, the respondent had admitted at interview that she took and used them (from some pre-signed prescriptions given to her for the practice's vaccination programme) because she was in extreme pain. She said that one of the doctors had said he would give her something temporarily but he had forgotten. She admitted to presenting the prescriptions at a chemist but leaving without any medicines when the pharmacist became suspicious and went to telephone the doctor. In completing the forms the respondent had used the names of two patients of the practice.

The police officer's evidence added that the respondent had been charged with one offence of theft, two offences of forging prescriptions and two offences of attempting to obtain medicines thereby. She had appeared in a Magistrates Court and pleaded guilty on all acounts. (Since the sentence of the court was not a prison sentence, fine or community service order the Committee proceedings could not proceed without the evidence referred to above.)

As indicated, the respondent did not appear at the hearing. She had, however, submitted two medical reports which indicated that (both in the past and at the time of the hearing) she had suffered from a painful back problem. She had only been employed by the practice for 1 month and no information was available about her previous work record. No mitigation was offered. The Committee was informed of previous offences involving prescriptions.

What lessons emerge from this case?

Which of the available decisions would you have chosen had you been a member of the Professional Conduct Committee?

CASE A19

A registered general nurse who had been employed as a practice nurse appeared before the Professional Conduct Committee as a result of an incident in the course of her professional work. The complaint had been brought by a woman patient of the practice and her husband.

The patient had only recently moved into the town to take a teaching post and had registered with the local group doctors' practice. Only a few weeks into her first term, at the age of 35 years, she realised to her pleasure that she was pregnant with a desperately wanted first pregnancy. At the end of a school day she went to the doctors' practice building to explain the situation. The only person she saw on that visit was the receptionist who heard what the patient had to say, took some notes and asked her to return the next morning at 10.00 AM.

The patient returned as instructed and was directed to the nurse's room. The nurse who became the subject of the case had arrived two hours earlier and, as usual, collected what was known as 'The Nurse's Book' from the receptionist. One of the entries in the book that morning, in the receptionist's writing, said 'Mrs X – Rubella'. The patient had not been seen by any of the doctors, nor had any prescription been written. At this practice an entry of the type indicated normally meant that an injection of live attenuated Rubella vaccine should be given. Without any explanation being given to the patient or any hint of consent the nurse hastily gave such an injection.

When it was realised what had happened the would-be parents were extremely angry and with justification. They decided that the pregnancy must be terminated. As a result of their complaints the nurse was dismissed but quickly obtained employment as a staff nurse in a general hospital. The aggrieved patient, feeling that the situation had not been adequately dealt with, brought a complaint alleging misconduct, and thus the case.

The respondent nurse admitted that the incident had happened exactly as described and was clearly distressed, remorseful and feeling very guilty about it. The investigation revealed that the practice was so devoid of any reasonable policies, procedures, practices or disciplines that an incident of this magnitude might well have happened any hour of any day. Quite clearly the respondent was not the only person responsible for that, since the doctors and her nurse colleague should not have allowed such a situation to exist. She was, however, accountable for her own actions.

She neither denied the facts or challenged the suggestion that those facts were misconduct in a professional sense. In mitigation she said that, when she joined the practice staff four years earlier, she was worried about much that she saw around her, but came to tolerate it because her nurse colleague and the doctors seemed untroubled. Further to that, she indicated that her hospital employers were fully aware of the incident when taking her on and produced written confirmation of this fact. She came across as a kind, caring person, but as one who was probably excessively compliant.

Had you been a member of the Professional Conduct Committee, would you have postponed judgment on the case and set some criteria to be satisfied, removed the respondent from the register, or closed the case with words of caution and counsel?

Identifying the principles within this case, ask yourself if anything like this could happen where you work.

CASE A20

Following her own admission to her nurse managers that she had struck a mentally handicapped resident on the thigh when seeking to protect another similar resident an enrolled nurse (for the mentally handicapped) was dismissed from employment, reported to the statutory bodies, and was referred by the investigating committee for a hearing before the Professional Conduct Committee.

Her written statement to the Investigating Committee was also put by her before the Professional Conduct Committee. It reads as follows:

'I had worked on the ward for just over a year prior to the incident. During that year I became disgusted with myself, the staff I worked with, and the system in which we worked; but mainly myself for not being able to do anything to change the system that I detested. Many of the problems resulted from staff shortages, but were also due to inadequate ward management, combined with low staff morale. All we could give our residents was basic nursing care, and that ineffectually. It was a soul-destroying experience.

New staff would arrived on the ward full of enthusiasm and good ideas. However, they soon became either disillusioned or cynical, like the rest of the staff. I would like to describe the conditions on the ward, to give you some idea as to the stresses for both residents and staff.

Everyday the same routine was followed. Everybody up, everybody to the bathroom, then everybody to the dining room for breakfast. It was one mad hectic rush, getting them up as quickly as possible, bathed, dressed and toileted, so that you could go on to the next one, and the next one subsequently. All this was done as quickly as possible. No time was available to allow the residents to do things for themselves at their own pace. The ward routine was regimented and on the whole inflexible, there being little or no margin for residents' personal choice.

It was very difficult to maintain a high standard of nursing, because this meant working slower, at the residents' pace. However, this would also result in other staff who worked at a faster pace completing more work, so leaving you feeling annoyed and guilty. Annoyed because in working faster, they had done everything for the residents, rather than letting them do the things they were capable of for themselves. Also I felt guilty working at the residents' pace, even though it resulted in residents doing things for themselves and me doing my job properly, as it also meant that other staff had more work to do. You could not win, continuity of a high standard of care was impossible. I felt torn between doing what was best for the individual resident, and seeing to everyone. Finding a balance between what was best for the individual and getting everything done was extremely difficult.

Any sort of suggested changes however slight were regarded suspiciously, from the sister down to the nursing assistants, because of what they would involve. However, in some respects, suggestions from student learners did carry more weight. On one occasion two learners went to the sister to complain and request that only one resident should be in the bathroom at one time. One bathroom and two toilets between eight people, is far from adequate, when all eight have to be got up, bathed, dressed, toileted and then have breakfast at the same time. Plus four more residents, who share one bathroom and toilet. All these twelve people had to be seen to in the space of two hours. People with handicaps ranging from severe mental and physical handicap, making them totally dependent on others; to those few who could talk and do things for themselves, but all needing close personal supervision. In this instance the change was eventually implemented. It did mean more work for the staff, but was much better for the residents. However, I was fairly certain that the sister, staff nurse and I, were the only ones to carry out this change, as other staff needed constant reminders.

Meal times were total *chaos*. We rarely had more than three or four staff per shift, who should have been divided between the two dining rooms at meal times. One dining room was given over to the more able residents, the other to those who needed extra assistance. So if there were enough domestics and housekeepers on duty they would see to the dining room for the more able, leaving the nursing staff to see to the other dining room. Even in these circumstances, sharing three or four staff between ten residents, who all needed some degree of supervision, from a prompt to eat to feeding completely, was very difficult. If you are feeding someone you need to concentrate on that person, so you can judge when they are ready for the next mouthful. Feeding a blind, deaf person whose head is continually moving is difficult enough on its own, without having to see to others. Between mouthfuls you are constantly looking around, making sure everyone is alright, and often getting side tracked. The person across the table is eating with their fingers, someone else has fallen asleep and numerous other interruptions such as these occur constantly throughout every meal. Meanwhile, the person you are supposed to be feeding has long since finished the last mouthful, or has gone off the idea of food.

To me this was a living nightmare which I was powerless to do anything about. Who could I tell? The sister was impervious to any suggested changes, and what could be done if I did take it higher? Telling tales about well-meaning, but overworked, demoralised colleagues did not appeal either. I had hoped that with an enthusiastic new director of nursing things would improve. On his first day in office, our cottage was down to two staff and we could get no help from other units, not even for a few hours. Two staff to twenty four residents – as long as you managed and said nothing management seemed happy. However, if you started complaining, all they wanted was a scapegoat. On this occasion I was deeply concerned and decided to ring the union. Within 15 minutes we had help, but the next day the nursing officer, who had been off the previous day, wanted to know who had caused trouble by ringing the union.

The conditions on the unit were in part due to the attitude of the new sister. She was reluctant to hold a staff meeting despite repeated requests during her first six months on the ward. She had previously worked on a children's unit and her attitude towards adults was exactly the same. She was opposed to them drinking any alcohol, although the strongest they drank was a half or two of shandy. She did not allow them more than 50 pence each to go out with, even over Christmas. This was despite the argument that it would barely cover the cost of one drink and a packet of crisps.

The day the incident took place I was worried about another resident. She looked as though she had given up and was going to die. She was eating and drinking very little, and showed no interest in anything. The staff nurse expressed the same opinion. Yes, I thought – we had done this to her, us and this rotten system. The residents walk around like jumble sales, their clothes are disgraceful. Anything you send to the launderette comes back ruined. Most of the residents are depressed or withdrawn. They spend most of their time in this dark, low ceilinged building, with only themselves and a bunch of miserable fed-up nursing staff for company.

Yes, I admit that I felt terrible the day of the incident as I had done for several months. I was also especially worried about the resident who was ill. Then to be slapped, kicked and spat at was the last straw. I could not walk away, another resident was receiving the same treatment. I was so frightened and sick and disgusted at myself for what I had done. I could not tell anyone what had happened, I could not sleep. There was nobody that I could turn to. As far as I am aware there is no procedure to cover a situation like this. I thought of going to the charge nurse on the next unit but was too frightened to.

In the end it was a relief to tell someone. I am very sorry for what took place. However, I feel that in many respects I was a victim of the extremely difficult circumstances that prevailed on the ward at that time. These circumstances were not under my control.

I only hope that the events following this incident will help to bring about some changes that will benefit both residents and staff, rather than being swept under the carpet and forgotten as it has been up to now.'

The two nurse managers called in evidence did not dispute the general accuracy of the enrolled nurse's statement.

Discuss the issues raised. Then consider whether, when set in its context which the letter well describes, you would consider the admitted striking to be misconduct. If your answer to that is 'Yes' what decision would you make? To take no further action – to postpone judgment for a stated period – or to remove from the register.

All the evidence received suggested that this young woman was a kind, competent, immensely caring nurse. The Committee clearly felt that all those things were true and that such qualities made her ideally suited to the care of the mentally handicapped. In contrast with that, however, the sheer fact that she cared so much seemed to make her vulnerable when working in a setting which made it extremely difficult to practise safely and well.

Finally apply the points made by this young enrolled nurse to reappraise your own practice and work setting.

CASE A21

A 25-year-old woman employed as a junior sister in an intensive therapy unit of a district general hospital appeared before the Professional Conduct Committee to face allegations which arose from the death of a patient in the unit.

The people who brought the allegations accepted that the patient's prognosis was poor in any case, but still believed that the circumstances raised serious questions about the safety of the practitioner who became the respondent.

In the intensive therapy unit in question it was discovered that the alarm on a particular type of positive pressure ventilator sounded with great frequency if it was used for mandatory assisted respiration at a rate of six respirations per minute or less. The matter was not drawn to the attention of the nurse managers of the hospital concerned, nor to the manufacturers of the equipment. Instead an *ad hoc* practice was developed in the unit (to which some of the medical staff including consultant anaesthetists were party) to switch off the alarm if the rate for which the machine was being set was six per minute or less.

This practice seemed to have been pursued without any unsavoury conse-quences for some months. However, on one particular day when there were three registered nurses on duty in the unit and only one patient, the patient's condition deteriorated to such a degree and in such a way that, had it not been switched off, the alarm would have sounded and called nursing staff to give urgent attention. The patient died.

At the Professional Conduct Committee the fact that the *ad hoc* practice of turning the alarm off had developed was not challenged – indeed, one consultant anaesthetist told the Committee that he had often come into the unit and heard the alarm sounding and took the necessary action to disconnect it because the problem was with the machine and not the patient. In support of such an action he argued that the alarm was meant to be an aid to human observation by a suitably qualified person and not a replacement for it.

The Committee had no difficulty in finding that the sister in question had turned off the alarm on the machine, but were faced with something of a dilemma in that one of the other trained staff on the ward at the time had subsequently performed required observations on the patient and had not turned it on again.

At the mitigation stage of the proceedings it became clear that the nurse in question had a previously unblemished record.

See yourself as a member of the Professional Conduct Committee. In particular, considering this case against the background of the UKCC Code of Professional Conduct, would you have regarded the proven action of this sister as misconduct in a professional sense? If so would you have then felt it necessary to remove her name from the part of the register for registered general nurses (the only part on which her name was) or not? In addition consider what lessons this case might have for your own practice and the settings in which you work.

CASE A22

The Professional Conduct Committee spent two days hearing and considering allegations against a registered mental nurse of 23 years standing who had been employed as a ward sister for over 15 years in the hospital in which she had trained and had continuously worked.

She appeared before the Committee with her registration status at stake because she was the subject of five allegations of professional misconduct arising out of incidents alleged to have occurred in the ward for which she was responsible, and at times when she was on duty. She was represented by an officer of her professional organisation.

The allegations were:

(1) That she failed to take action against a nursing assistant when he escorted two male patients clad only in pyjama jackets through the ward in the presence of female patients.

(2) That she similarly failed to take action when the same person carried a naked male patient through the ward in the presence of female patients.

(3) That she similarly failed to take action when the same person deliberately put shaving foam into the mouth of the patient.

(4) That she acted in a way prejudicial to the well-being and welfare of a patient in her care by remarking to the night staff that they were not to worry if a

patient foamed at the mouth, he was not having a fit but had had his mouth washed out with soap.

(5) That she failed to maintain a proper professional attitude by making the remark referred to in (4).

The incidents were alleged to have occurred over a four-month period. The ward was a mixed sex psychogeriatic ward. The layout was not really appropriate for an integrated ward, since there was one dormitory housing male and female elderly patients, and screens or curtains were in fairly short supply. Also there were problems in respect of adequacy of supply of linen and patients' clothing. The ward seemed adequately staffed.

Evidence in respect of the charges (1) and (2) came from a former staff nurse at the hospital who, at the time of the hearing, was working in the community. He described two incidents when a particular nursing assistant took the actions referred to in the charges at a time when the sister was in the ward. While he believed she probably observed those incidents and expressed the view that it would have been difficult for her not to have been aware of them since he (the staff nurse) had remonstrated with the nursing assistant, he quite honestly stated that he could not testify that the sister did see these incidents.

Evidence in respect of the third charge came from an enrolled nurse and several nursing assistants who had gathered in the day room where the patient in question was being shaved by the nursing assistant who featured in several of the charges.

They explained how, on realising what he was doing to the patient, they reacted angrily and noisily, and had no doubt that the sister, who was in the kitchen which had an open hatch linking it to the day room, on hearing the altercation, put her head through the hatch, clearly saw what was going on, but then withdrew into the kitchen and then took no subsequent action. Some of the same witnesses provided evidence in respect of charges (4) and (5), both in respect of the application of soap from a bar at the ward sink to the patient's mouth, and of the remark to the night staff. It should be noted that, in respect of evidence, the standard of proof that the Committee must have before they find any charges proved is that they are satisfied beyond reasonable doubt that the incidents occurred.

At the conclusion of evidence in support of the charges the respondent's representative used the opportunity provided by the law to make certain submissions. First she submitted that the evidence was not such that the Committee would be able to find the facts proved, and second that those facts could not constitute misconduct in a professional sense. The Committee considered those matters in camera, and then announced in public their agreement with the first submission in respect of charges (1) and (2) only, but their rejection of both submissions in respect of charges (3), (4) and (5).

This meant that the respondent had to provide a defence against three charges, but for this purpose the male nursing assistant who had been the subject of the shaving incident, together with two members of night staff were called. At the end of that evidence the Committee again retired into camera, and subsequently announced in public that they found the facts alleged in charges (3), (4) and (5) proved to their satisfaction. Further argument was submitted as to why they should not be considered misconduct, but the Committee found them to be such.

In the mitigation/aggravation stage that followed it emerged that, with the exception of the period when the nursing assistant in question was on the ward, the sister had apparently run that ward to the satisfaction of her employers for a long period of time. Even the staff who had testified against her in support of the charges had been amazed at her failure to take action in respect of the shaving foam incident. A substantial number of testimonials were produced in support of her remaining on the register from medical, nursing and social work staff, and others from a priest and a patient's relative. She had not been dismissed as a result of the incident, but had been the subject of some local discipline and had subsequently moved to another ward where again her performance was regarded as highly satisfactory.

Try to put yourself into the position of the five members who constituted the Committee. On the one hand you have a sister of long experience in one institution whose standard of practice over most of that time seems to have been exemplary. On the other hand you have found it proved that, on two certain occasions during a two-month period, she appeared to condone by her own inaction some appalling ill treatment of an elderly and highly dependent patient, and made it the subject of remarks which were deemed both prejudicial to the well-being of the patient and contrary to proper professional attitudes.

Given all these circumstances would you have decided to postpone judgment for a stated period, or to remove this ward sister from the register and thus prevent her practising, or take no further action other than to draw her attention to the expectations of her listed in the Code of Professional Conduct? Ask yourself also whether such things might possibly be happening in the place in which you work or for which you have a management responsibility.

CASE A23

A 48-year-old woman appeared before the Professional Conduct Committee following an incident during the course of her professional work as a registered midwife some months earlier. She had come to midwifery at a mature age as a direct entrant (i.e. with no previous nursing qualifications), but at the time of the incident had nine years experience as a midwife.

She was employed as a community midwife in a large city, and had a student midwife attached (her first after three years without). The charges she faced arose from allegations that she failed to urgently summon medical aid when there was evidence of likely fetal distress, and failed to adequately supervise a student midwife (approximately 2 months in training).

The circumstances were as follows. The community midwives used a community/general practitioner unit for the deliveries for which they had a responsibility. It was located at a hospital, immediately next to and only divided by an unlocked door from the consultant obstetrics unit. One night, at about 12.15 AM, the midwife had a call from the hospital to say that a 19-year-old woman had arrived at the community midwifery unit, and was one of that midwife's patients. The midwife immediately telephoned her new student (whom she had not met) and asked her to travel to the unit. The midwife arrived at approximately 12.50 AM, five minutes before her student. She found that the patient was one who had made several local house moves in a short time, had never been found at home by the midwife when visiting, and had received no antenatal care. During the five minutes before the student arrived the midwife, with a little difficulty, located a fetal heart, which she did not record but subsequently described as 'soft but regular'. (The hospital midwife who called her to this unexpected patient had checked when the patient arrived, and she had recorded the fetal heart as 'strong'.)

When the student arrived the midwife requested her to go through the required admission and examination procedure. One of her first actions was to take the patient's blood pressure, which she found to be significantly raised, especially the diastolic pressure. The student expressed concern at the finding which she recorded, but it was not checked, and she was told to continue with her examination. She could not find a fetal heart but was told that the midwife had with difficulty. The student was asked if she had attached fetal scalp electrodes before, and replied that she had only seen it done. She was told to apply electrodes after completing a vaginal examination.

She tried her best to comply with the instruction, and eventually succeeded after some difficulty, the patient being in some distress and preferring to lie on her side. Some nine minutes after the scalp electrodes had been attached the student observed the recording was not being properly made, not least because the paper was 'burning', but her concern seemed not to be shared or understood. The midwife seemed content with the figures flashing on the visual indicator, of which she had no record in the absence of a proper reading. After a further slight delay, the student took it on herself to go to seek aid at the consultant unit, whence she returned with a midwifery sister. The sister immediately saw that the equipment was not properly set up in that the paper roll was not aligned or mounted on the sprocket holes. She corrected this, checked and corrected the attachment of the electrodes and (having observed the recording then showing) said to the midwife 'I would call for medical assistance urgently if I were you!' It was then approximately 1.25 AM.

The sister departed, and the midwife told the student to continue and complete her admission procedures. These were eventually completed just before 1.45 AM, at which time the fetal heart recording was showing cause for real concern, and the blood pressure taken by the student indicated a further increase. Only then, with the admission/examination procedures complete in her view, did the midwife go to call the patient's general practitioner by telephone. She found that his calls were redirected to a deputising service, to whom she then spoke. They said the only doctor on duty with obstetric experience was engaged in another part of the city, and would not be free to leave there until about 2.10 AM, and would arrive at approx. 2.30 AM.

On her return to the ward where the patient was in the care of the student, the midwife found the situation deteriorating further. She telephoned the deputising service again, and they told her they would arrange a police escort to get the doctor there in the minimum of time.

Several minutes later (by now approximately 2.05 AM) there was a sudden prolapse of the cord. The student's immediate reaction was to apply pressure to the fetal head to prevent it constricting the cord. The midwife said that she left her with the patient, went through the door to the consultant unit, and shouted 'prolapsed cord' very loudly, several times. The sister who had visited earlier, and her senior colleague rushed to the patient. They quickly summed up the situation, summoned 'hospital medical aid' (which was on call in the unit), and moved the patient. Within minutes a Caesarian section had been performed.

Unfortunately the patient was delivered of a fresh male stillbirth.

The evidence to prove that the sequence of events had been as described came from the student, sister, and nursing officer, and from the midwife herself. She denied the charges, though agreeing to the sequence of events. She insisted that they had done the right things in the right order, and that she summoned medical aid as soon as the admission procedures were completed. The Committee found the facts proved and considered them misconduct. Would you have agreed?

At the mitigation stage it emerged that there was considerable antipathy between the midwifery staff of the consultant unit and the community midwives who used the other unit. The midwife's manager said that the midwife only rarely took the in-service training opportunities provided, and that she had required counselling on the subject of student supervision on a number of occasions, culminating in the removal of students for a significant period.

You are the Professional Conduct Committee. What will you do?

CASE A24

A very experienced community midwife appeared before the Professional Conduct Committee charged with misconduct arising from a sequence of failures to take appropriate action when called to attend upon a 16-year-old new mother suffering a postpartum haemorrhage several days after transfer home from hospital.

The birth/postnatal period had been uneventful, and mother and baby were transferred home to the small inner-city flat where she lived with the 18-year-old boyfriend who was the father of the baby.

On the ninth day after delivery he returned home at 5.45 PM where he found that the baby's mother was lying on the bed. She was doing so because she had bled slightly and was uncertain about whether that was normal or not. He proceeded with preparing a meal and caring for the baby. After resting on the bed for some time she needed to go to the toilet, but on standing was shocked by the fact that a large blood clot (she said the size of an orange) fell on to the rug. She quickly got back to bed. Over the next hour she produced large clots with increasing frequency. The boyfriend gathered them up and kept them in a line of plastic bags because he was unsure what else to do with them.

At the end of that hour they agreed that this could not be normal, and that he should telephone the number which they had been given to obtain a midwife. He managed to find a telephone which had not been vandalised and made a call to the number he had been given which proved to be the emergency bed service of a hospital which operated a message receiving and forwarding service. Records made available to the Committee indicated the accuracy of the message the boyfriend had conveyed and of that which had been passed on to the midwife (who became the subject of this case) within minutes.

She arrived at the flat an hour after the call was made. She was not known to the family. According to the evidence of the young mother and father, the midwife immediately expressed her displeasure that the mother was on a low divan bed since she had difficulty in bending. Their evidence also indicated that, apart from placing a tentative hand on the abdomen by way of examination and assisting him to place an incontinence pad underneath her, the midwife did no active work. Instead she gave the father instructions about the continuing cleaning up and clot gathering, interfering only to ask for a chair to be brought so that she could sit rather than stand. During this period of the evening, when going for water and other things, he opened the door to various members of the family who were calling, all of whom gathered in the kitchen when told the midwife was present.

The evidence of the two young people went on to indicate that during this period the midwife seemed to be thinking aloud about whether she should call an ambulance or not, and said that she would have to do so if the mother was having a haemorrhage but that was not the case. Suddenly she left the flat without saying where she was going or what she was going to do.

By now, drinking tea in the kitchen, were the girl's father, stepbrother and the latter's wife (who happened to be a nurse/midwife and herself 12 days overdue for the expected delivery of her own first child). The midwife having disappeared, this pregnant relative went to see the young mother and was extremely disturbed about the situation which she found. She was not in current employment as a midwife and was not equipped as the respondent midwife would have been with appropriate drugs. She sought to rub up a contraction, meanwhile urging the various members of the family to go and call an ambulance. At first they were reluctant to do this because they felt that the midwife may have gone to do so and they did not want to upset her. As the situation further deteriorated her insistence prevailed and they called an ambulance at approximately 9.30 PM from a phonebox in a nearby public house and hastily returned to the flat. An ambulance arrived outside the block of flats a few minutes later, and coincidentally the midwife pulled up in her car. The ambulance staff were unhappy about the situation which they found as they entered the flat and (it would appear) pushed the respondent midwife aside in order to take the young mother to hospital without any delay. The father went in the ambulance with her but the midwife did not. On her arrival at the accident and emergency department of a nearby major hospital several minutes later she was found to be seriously ill. Blood was taken for cross-matching and an IV infusion commenced. The doctor who treated her there was called in evidence, as was the senior registrar in obstetrics who took the case over. The latter said it was the worst postpartum haemorrhage he had seen. An urgent evacuation of retained products was performed and several units of blood given. The patient recovered satisfactorily.

Other witnesses included a midwifery sister from the hospital to which the patient was taken and a general practitioner of the group practice of which she was a patient. The hospital midwifery sister described how, at a time coincident with the respondent midwife's absence from the flat, that midwife had appeared in the obstetric unit asking her questions. She knew her to be a community midwife of long standing, and was surprised that she was asking about the circumstances in which you call an ambulance or the emergency obstetric unit or insist that the ambulance you are calling have IV infusion equipment. She said she did not think the midwife could be talking about a patient who was somewhere bleeding at that moment because she would have been with the patient rather than in the unit talking with her. The GP told how the respondent had telephoned him from the hospital (the time sequence would suggest after the conversation with the midwifery sister). She did not ask him to call, but seemed to have again gone into the question about the circumstances in which you call for which type of assistance. He was left sufficiently confused that he felt the safest thing to do was to call on the patient. He arrived at the flat shortly after the patient had been taken to hospital. He was able to hear something of the sequence of events from the members of the family who remained in the flat and to form an assessment of the volume of blood loss by seeing the quite large collection of plastic bags containing clots and also quantities of blood soaked linen and pads, etc. He communicated his conclusions to the obstetric unit.

The respondent denied the allegations in respect of her failure but all matters alleged were proved to the satisfaction of the Committee. It also regarded them as misconduct in a professional sense. Consider whether you would have agreed with them on the latter point.

At the mitigation stage, through her representative, the midwife continued to insist that the charges would have been appropriate and would have amounted to misconduct had the patient been having a postpartum haemorrhage, but continued to insist that this was not the case. She gave no alternative explanation for the significant blood loss over several hours and seemed unmoved by the evidence of the three doctors who were called. Contrary to the situation in many cases involving midwives of long experience her representative produced no written evidence from previous grateful patients about her competence as a practitioner. This may have been more a failure on his part than on hers.

Consider this case and decide whether, in respect of the now proven misconduct, you will decide to postpone judgment for a period, or to remove the respondent from the register as a midwife (the only part of the register on which her name is found) or take no action other than to express some words of caution and advice. Consider also whether any lessons emerge which you might apply to your own practice and work setting.

CASE A25

A 35-year-old enrolled nurse was the subject of charges before the Professional Conduct Committee to the effect that he was guilty of misconduct, having (1) drunk alcohol while on night duty, and (2) slept in a patient's bed.

The respondent did not attend the hearing, which therefore commenced with evidence being given of the formal notice of the enquiry having been delivered to his registered address. The respondent had not responded to a request for a statement or explanation for the Investigating Committee, so no evidence was available as to his response to the allegations made against him.

The incidents were alleged to have occurred at night in a long-stay ward of a large psychiatric hospital. The respondent had been the only member of the nursing staff on duty with 32 patients. A night sister normally visited the ward on three occasions during the night. She had visited twice (at approximately 8.30 PM and 12.30 AM) and found things quiet and normal. She then injured an ankle, and did not complete a third round. Instead she sought to make contact by telephone, but this was not successful, and shortly before the end of the shift sent an enrolled nurse from another ward to collect the report she required.

That nurse arrived ten minutes before the shift handover, and encountered the day charge nurse who had arrived several minutes earlier. As he arrived the telephone in the ward office was ringing. He answered it and received a request for the night nurse. He began to look for the respondent, and was joined in his search by the other enrolled nurse when she arrived. Together, they looked in offices, kitchen, toilets, bathrooms and cupboards without success.

At this stage a patient asked if they were looking for the night nurse. On being told 'Yes' the patient gestured, and said 'He's down there in bed'. They went down the dormitory as directed, and were expecting that (if true) it would be an otherwise empty bed. They were, therefore, surprised to find the nurse in an occupied bed. The charge nurse described the patient as 'looking like a bird whose nest had been invaded', and reported him as saying that he didn't mind very much but the beds were a bit narrow for two! In evidence to the Committee the charge nurse and enrolled nurse described how they found the respondent deeply asleep, and how they had to shout and shake him to wake him. When they eventually succeeded he swung his legs over the side of the bed, at which stage they realised that he was clad only in underpants. There was an unintended piece of humour in the evidence at this stage when the charge nurse in answer to a question as to what he then said to the respondent, replied 'I told him he was wanted on the telephone'.

This matter was reported to the responsible managers as a result of which the director of nursing services planned to contact the respondent nurse later in the day to advise him of his suspension from duty pending enquiries. However, before the DNS could take that action the respondent nurse arrived at the hospital in the late morning and insisted on seeing him. The DNS in evidence explained that he had counselled the respondent to be accompanied for the interview but he declined. The DNS also indicated that he had tried his best to warn him of the danger of saying anything self-incriminating, and to at least allow him time to call an observer. However, this was not allowed to happen.

The DNS testified that the respondent blurted out that he had been having serious personal/domestic problems which had reached a peak the previous day, and had brought a bottle of vodka with him when he came on duty. After the night sister's second round he had steadily consumed the vodka over a 2-hour period. At about 2.45 AM he encountered a patient who had said he looked tired and suggested that he go to bed for a while. Unwisely he did this, thinking he was using a vacant bed. He knew no more until woken by the charge nurse at 6.55 AM. Having said all that he handed in his written resignation and left.

Given that evidence of three witnesses would you find the facts proved? If 'Yes' would you consider them misconduct in a professional sense? If 'Yes' what would be your judgment? There was no evidence in mitigation from the respondent. The DNS indicated he had been a satisfactory employee for four years, and they had not been aware of him having any special problems.

What cautionary tales emerge from this case?

Chapter 13

Professional Accountability Case Studies: 'Aspects of Accountability'

A short series of studies illustrating dilemmas experienced by practitioners in the course of their professional practice.

The reader who has considered carefully the information and arguments provided in Chapters 1, 2, 5 and 9 should now be equipped to consider the following studies and to arrive at some personal conclusions.

Unlike the cases in Chapter 13, these studies have not been the subject of any committee consideration, since no complaint has been made to the profession's regulatory body about any nurse, midwife or health visitor involved. They ask you to put yourself in the shoes of the person whose actual dilemma each study records and to consider what your answers to the following two questions would be:

(1) What do you consider to be the correct professional response in this situation?
(2) What do you think you would actually have done?

Comments on the cases are provided in Appendix 4. I recommend that reference be made to that section only after each study has been read, considered and discussed.

STUDY B1

A practice nurse employed by a large GP practice went home from work one day to find that her house had been broken into and possessions to the value of about £4000 stolen. One of the missing items was a very unusual and distinctive bracelet of great sentimental value and a monetary value of some £400.

Three months later, when this nurse was on duty in the practice, a woman patient was directed to her room for some treatment. The nurse immediately noticed that the patient was wearing a bracelet exactly like that stolen from her home. The nurse was taken aback by this, but, with great self-control, said how very unusual the bracelet was and how much she admired it. The patient's response was to say 'Yes, it is lovely isn't it. I was given it as a present about 12 weeks ago.' There was no suggestion of guilt or anxiety in this response.

The nurse's suspicions were aroused by this response. What should she do? Her financial loss is being met by her insurers, but she naturally feels aggrieved by the invasion of her home and the theft. On the one hand, the woman may have been given the bracelet by someone who had purchased it through proper channels. On the other hand, to go to the police may lead to those responsible for this and other burglaries. It is clear that the police could do nothing if she does not disclose the patient's name and address, but that would be a breach of confidentiality. Could she justify that action?

STUDY B2

A nurse applied for and was appointed to a post as the nursing officer for a neurosurgical unit of three wards. The vacancy had been created by the promotion of the former post holder to a more senior nursing management position. The new nursing officer was new to this health authority. Her line manager was the person into whose former post she had stepped.

Almost immediately the nursing officer began to observe that, on all the wards in the unit, although the trained nursing staff was adequate, all the major nursing care, including such activities as neurological observations, the care of patients in the immediate postoperative phase and the eye care of patients newly admitted with cranial injuries was performed by unqualified staff working unsupervised.

Concerned at what she regarded as completely unnecessary and improper delegation, the new nursing officer raised the matter in a meeting with all the ward sisters (all of whom had been in post for a substantial period of time) and was surprised that the reaction she received from them was first to state that they could see nothing wrong and second to point out that the previous nursing officer knew all about it and that her superiors had demonstrated confidence in her by promoting her. Disturbed by this reaction, the nursing officer sought to raise the matter in a diplomatic way with her predecessor/line manager, only to receive a fairly similar response.

STUDY B3

The combination of limited financial resources and increasing problems of recruitment of registered nurses has led a health authority to conduct a reappraisal of its policies for staffing at night.

One of the decisions made and announced is that, when the operating theatres are not in action during the night, the theatre nursing staff will be redeployed. The reaction of the theatre staff to this is not to be particularly worried, since in this large city general hospital the operating theatres are busy almost every night and, if they were allocated elsewhere, they would always be placed in support of other staff as the prospect would always exist of their recall to theatre if emergencies arose. They simply stated their expectation on this point to their managers and were told nothing to disillusion them.

Some weeks later, quite exceptionally, the operating theatre was not in action three hours into the night shift. The senior staff nurse on theatre duty was suddenly instructed to go to take charge of a large, busy paediatric ward in which there were a number of very ill children. She was told by the night sister that the unqualified staff on the ward would tell her about the patients as she did not have time to go to the ward herself.

Although she has been a registered nurse for 12 years the theatre staff nurse has worked only in operating theatres for all of those 12 years. She has had no ward experience since registration and had only eight weeks allocation to a paediatric ward when a student nurse.

STUDY B4

A nurse accepts appointment as a clinical specialist for breast and stoma care and finds she has to work in association with three surgeons who perform breast surgery. She quickly comes to realise that the first surgeon is open and honest with the patients and performs surgery strictly in accordance with what he finds to be necessary. She also realises that the second surgeon, while only personally performing radical mastectomy for malignant conditions, is open and honest about it when seeking consent and places no obstacle in the way of patients who wish to seek a second opinion before agreeing to what they see as mutilating surgery. She has no problems about the attitudes manifested by those two surgeons.

The nurse observes, however, over a course of several months, that the third surgeon, in seeking consent for the operation, always told the patient that it was almost certain that he would have to remove a small lump only, but who, once in the operating room always performed radical mastectomy and sometimes referred to the patient as being another one he had misled.

Having come to this realisation, what should the nurse do? What key elements of her role become relevant?

If she worries about it but does nothing for several further weeks, what should she do when a patient of the third surgeon, having just signed a consent form, comes to the nurse saying how relieved she is to have been told that almost certainly she will only have a little lump removed?

STUDY B5

A staff nurse employed in a ward of a psychiatric hospital has in her care a compulsorily detained young adult female patient. The hospital has no evidence of the patient having parents, guardians or other relatives.

The medical and nursing staff are of the opinion that, both within the hospital and out in the nearby town where she is known to be meeting some former patients of the hospital, her behaviour is very promiscuous.

Suddenly a junior doctor declares that, since the patient is not in a position to give consent were she asked, and since there is no-one else from whom to seek consent, he is going to take some blood for an HIV test without consent and that he requires the staff nurse's assistance.

The staff nurse is troubled about this from legal, ethical and practical standpoints. What repercussions might there be one way or the other?

STUDY B6

A staff nurse who had been employed in an expensive private nursing home for just a few weeks (this being her return to nursing after a 12-year break) came on duty one day and was asked, with some unqualified staff, to move the patients, their beds, associated furniture and property from their present location to a room in an annexe attached to the main building. This she did, noticing that the room (in a part of the building she had not previously entered) was less accessible and of a less satisfactory standard than the rooms in the main building and was at the top of some steep, narrow stairs. Some other patients were accommodated in other rooms in this annexe. Shortly afterwards she noticed that the room the patients had vacated had been equipped with a television set and armchairs.

Later that same day, while still on duty, she became aware that a professional team from the health authority were coming on an announced visit of inspection. The team conducted their visit while she was still on duty. They seemed satisfied with what they saw, and overheard comments indicated that they had seen the number of patients for which the home had a registration certificate. The staff nurse realised that the inspection team had not been taken beyond the door that led into the annexe. She went off duty a little troubled. When she returned to duty the next morning the two patients she had moved were back in the room that, for the period of the inspection, had become a lounge and TV room. Other patients were still in the annexe room.

STUDY B7

Two young registered nurses employed in a paediatric unit became concerned when two consultant anaesthetists were seen to be prescribing drugs for premedication for children which were far in excess of anything previously prescribed for the purpose. Having first spoken to the ward sister and discovering that she shared their concern but did not believe it to be her place to question the doctors, they raised their concerns with the anaesthetists and were told by them that they were engaged in a research project, that it would be alright and that they would bear the full responsibility.

Still concerned, realising from the manufacturer's literature that the quantities being prescribed were often ten or more times the recommended maximum dose (for children of the body weight involved), the nurses (through one of their number) telephoned the manufacturers. The technical spokesman of the firm expressed his horror at what he had been told, but declined to confirm his concern in writing.

Enquiries which the nurses directed to the nurse member of the local ethical committee revealed that no such research project had been before the committee for approval.

STUDY B8

A staff nurse and an enrolled nurse, who were very good friends both in work and outside of work, were on night duty on a children's medical ward. During their period of duty a six-year-old patient went into a hypoglycaemic coma and was transferred to the intensive care unit of the same hospital. Immediately after the patient's transfer the staff nurse told the enrolled nurse that she (the staff nurse) had miscalculated and administered a much larger dose of insulin than had been prescribed by the doctor. The staff nurse said that she had not reported this mistake and that she did not intend to do so. She told the enrolled nurse not to report it as she was admitting this mistake to her in confidence and it would be unethical if the enrolled nurse broke this confidence.

STUDY B9

A team of community psychiatric nurses have been working for a health authority for some time and to the apparent satisfaction of their patients, their nursing managers, the general practitioners (who referred them most of their patients and with whom they worked closely) and the consultant psychiatrists. In completing claims for their travelling expenses they have (without objection) stated only the general part of the town visited but not the name of the patient or the exact address. They have always been willing to show their work diaries and (if necessary) their records to their immediate nurse manager if he wished to do a sample check of their claims since they properly regarded him as bound by the same professional ethic as themselves.

A new director of nursing has now taken up post and insists that all community nursing staff, of whatever speciality, must give the full names and exact addresses of all patients or clients visited, that they will not be paid their travelling expenses if they do not comply and that non-compliance will meet with disciplinary action.

The community psychiatric nurses are concerned at this ruling on principle. Their concern is made greater by the fact that some of their patients, through GP referral, are employees of the health authority whose confidentiality they do not wish to breach, even under orders.

STUDY B10

In the course of private conversastion with an informal patient in a psychiatric unit a charge nurse was informed by that patient that, for a period of time in the recent past, he had sexually abused two young girls who were his nieces.

Concerned about the information he now possessed and being also concerned at the possibility of further such abuse directed to the same or other children, the charge nurse shared the information now in his possession with his immediate nurse manager.

His own professional superior told him that, as soon as such information began to emerge, he should have drawn the conversation to a close and withdrawn from the situation, since his own position might become compromised. The charge nurse, however, found that the situation was not as simple as that, since, with no indication of what might be to come, the patient suddenly blurted out the full facts. In any event, he was far from convinced about the validity of the advice he was being given which was to the effect that he should do nothing.

STUDY B11

A sister of an intensive therapy unit of an NHS district general hospital observed that, with reasonable frequency, patients were transferred in from a local private hospital following major surgery in the course of which complications had developed which were seemingly beyond the capacity of that private hospital.

She was generally worried about this. Her concern rose to a new level, however, as a result of one such case.

The notes received with a 74-year-old patient were sketchy, but revealed that he had been admitted to the private hospital for a prostatectomy and had (shortly after admission) been subjected to some form of screening procedure. As a result he had been told (so he subsequently told the sister in ITU) he had some evidence of early gall bladder disease, that it would be wise to have the matter dealt with by cholecystectomy and that it could be done while he was anaesthetised for the prostatectomy. His consent was given.

It also became apparent from the limited notice that, when the prostatic bed was being irrigated, the patient went into ventricular failure and needed urgent resuscitative action. It was believed that absorption of some of the irrigating fluid through an unintended cut in the bladder may have been instrumental in causing the collapse.

The patient having been resuscitated, the operating team had then proceeded to perform the cholecystectomy. At the end of this second operation the patient was seriously ill and, as indicated above, was transferred to the ITU of the district general hospital.

The patient regained consciousness and was able to converse with the nursing staff in a lucid manner. During this period he said enough to convince the sister that he had experienced no symptoms of gall bladder disease and was surprised to be told of the need for a cholecystectomy.

The patient deteriorated rapidly and died a few days later. The sister realised that he was the third patient to be transferred into ITU from this private hospital over just three or four months to refer to operations having been performed for asymptomatic and non-malignant conditions and it worried her greatly.

STUDY B12

A nursing officer of a psychiatric unit was faced with a dilemma which was shared by some of the charge nurses within the unit of which he was the nurse manager.

The unit contained one 'secure' locked ward but also a number of wards which were not locked.

There were some patients on the unlocked wards whose condition and behaviour gave cause for serious concern. The psychiatrists, however, were reluctant to use their powers under the Mental Health Act to compulsorily detain these patients as they felt that to do so 'stigmatises' them. These patients therefore remained in the unlocked wards where staffing levels and mix were geared to expectations of the anticipated type of occupants.

However, the same psychiatrists stated their requirement that the same patients, accommodated as informal patients in unlocked wards, must be 'specialled'. This they stated as meaning a one to one nurse/patient contact at all times, the nurse always to remain 'within arm's length' of the patient.

STUDY B13

A clinical nurse manager has found himself under pressure to reduce staffing to a level required by his managers to meet their financial targets. He takes such steps as he believes to be consistent with (just) satisfying the standards for the elderly mentally infirm unit developed at the requirement of the health authority and approved by its members, but is still required by his senior managers to do more.

Were he to do so it is manifestly obvious to him, however, that those standards could not possibly be satisfied with a further reduced staffing while the number of patients remains the same. He is convinced that standards of care will inevitably be jeopardised, staff morale suffer with consequent increases in sickness/absence and patients placed at risk. The senior managers show no interest in reducing the workload but demand further reduction in pay costs and are seemingly not interested in the evidence to support his contention that the authority's own newly approved and publicised standards will not be met.

This manager has received comprehensive information from the sisters/ charge nurses of the three wards in the unit and has made his case in articulate, well documented form, but to no avail. He is now feeling that he is putting his job in jeopardy.

STUDY B14

A nurse manager contacted the UKCC to talk through the issues raised for the nursing staff of a ward by a decision of the medical staff in respect of one long-term patient.

The particular patient had been admitted two years earlier following a major road accident. He had been deeply unconscious throughout the time, but had been breathing without assisted ventilation. As a result of excellent nursing and an effective regime of nasogastric tube feeding recommended by a dietitian, the patient had, in all other respects, remained in excellent physical shape and had not lost weight. Indeed, a casual visitor to the ward could well assume that he was a generally healthy man of about 35 years of age who had a transient problem requiring a nasogastric tube and who was enjoying a good sleep.

The dilemma had arisen because the senior medical staff, after long and careful deliberation, had decided that there was no prospect of a cure and that feeding should cease, water being the only liquid to be provided via the tube, and that he be allowed to die. The relatives had been consulted and had agreed with the decision, but their agreement has no standing in law.

For some of the nurses who had been on the ward throughout this period the decision caused concern. The man, although unconscious, had become part of their collective life. His condition was only as good as it was because of the quality and quantity of nursing care they had provided. But now they were to starve him and see him fade and wither before their eyes, while they still provided care, until he died. Some wondered if this decision was based on economic factors rather than genuine medical reasons. While accepting the basic logic of the medical decision, the nurses were to be left with the steadily occurring consequences of it every minute of every day. Some nurses expressed the view that it would be better to remove the tube immediately. Some nurses felt unable to be party to further care under these circumstances and stated this to their nurse manager.

STUDY B15

A community psychiatric nurse found herself faced with a considerable dilemma relating to confidentiality arising out of her practice.

One of her clients was known by her to have been banned from driving following convictions for driving with a blood alcohol substantially above the limit and driving while uninsured. These offences and the resulting convictions had occurred before she became the nurse allocated to his case. As a result of her involvement she was also aware that he was receiving medication which might impair his judgment and make driving inadvisable.

She had felt for some time that she was developing a good and potentially therapeutic relationship with this client and had high hopes that it might succeed in achieving the breakthrough that a previous episode of inpatient treatment failed to achieve. The dilemma had arisen, however, because the nurse had now seen the client driving a car alone on a number of occasions in the busy town in which they both live.

What should the nurse do? On the one hand she recognises the risk of possible serious injury to her client or other people if he is involved in an accident because she has not informed the police. On the other hand she realises that if she does so inform, the therapeutic relationship which she believes to be developing with a chance of genuine progress will be shattered and any subsequent treatment programme rendered more difficult. She has quietly mentioned to him that she has seen him driving, but it has not achieved the change she hoped for.

Appendix 1

'With a view to removal from the register. . .?'

INTRODUCTION

(1) Section 12 of the Nurses, Midwives and Health Visitors Act, 1979, requires the United Kingdom Central Council for Nursing, Midwifery and Health Visiting (abbreviated to UKCC and referred to as the Council) to make statutory rules (that is, to prepare subordinate law for approval by senior Government law officers) governing the circumstances and the means by which a person's name may be removed from the register.

(2) This subordinate law (the Professional Conduct Rules) is set out in Statutory Instrument 1987 No. 2156 for England, Wales and Scotland and Statutory Instrument 1987 No. 473 for Northern Ireland.

(3) These rules require the Council to:

- assemble committees of its members to consider allegations of misconduct made against persons whose names appear on its register. Any such committee is a Professional Conduct Committee;
- set up two committees drawn from its members (the Panel of Screeners and the Health Committee) to consider allegations that the fitness to practise of persons identified in its register may be seriously impaired by illness.

(4) The purpose of a Professional Conduct Committee hearing is:

- to hear evidence under oath and to decide whether matters alleged are proved;
- to consider proven facts in context and decide whether, in professional terms, they constitute misconduct;
- to hear information about the respondent's previous history, and any submissions in mitigation of the proven misconduct;
- to decide whether the name of the practitioner should be removed from the register in the interests of patients and clients.

(5) The purpose of the consideration of documents by the Panel of Screeners and the Health Committee hearing is to decide:

- whether the practitioner's fitness to practise is impaired by physical or mental illness;
- whether the degree of impairment is so serious that, given the interest of patients/ clients, the practitioner should be removed from the register.

(6) However, the purpose of these committee proceedings is not:

- to punish the practitioner appearing before the committee (though the person

137

whose name is removed may so interpret a decision of removal from the register);
- to provide an employer with grounds to dismiss the practitioner;
- to provide an employer with an additional avenue of complaint to use when an appeal against dismissal has been upheld.

(7) Section two of this document, together with Annexe A, provides a brief explanation of the process of investigation, hearing and judgment of allegations of misconduct. It also provides information (based on Professional Conduct Committee decisions during the period 1984–1989) about categories of offence which have often led to removal from the register, and those which have not usually resulted in use of that sanction.

(8) Section three of this document, together with Annexe B, provides a brief explanation of the process of assembling medical and other relevant information, consideration by the Panel of Screeners, hearing before the Health Committee and judgment of allegations of unfitness to practise due to illness. It also provides information about categories of illness which often lead to removal from the register.

COMPLAINTS ALLEGING MISCONDUCT

Who can forward complaints alleging misconduct?

(9) It is any person's right to allege that the actions or omissions of a registered nurse, midwife or health visitor constitute misconduct in a professional sense, and call into question her continued registration status.

(10) This right equally applies to any employee of an organisation providing health care as much as to any other private citizen. Where the employee is a registered nurse, midwife or health visitor, there are circumstances in which that right becomes a duty.

When should a complaint be made?

(11) Where the complaint arises from an incident associated with the practitioner's professional practice, which is not and has not been the subject of criminal proceedings, it should be reported as soon as possible. This helps to ensure that the incident will be fresh in the memories of potential witnesses and also that those witnesses will still be readily available. If a matter is serious enough to warrant an allegation of misconduct, it should be reported immediately rather than eventually.

(12) The formal report of a complaint alleging misconduct should not be delayed pending the completion of employment appeal procedures.

(13) Cases resulting from conviction in criminal courts should be reported as described in 15.

How are complaints made?

(14) Many complaints alleging misconduct follow criminal court hearings where guilt has been proved. There are well established systems for a wide range of criminal findings to be reported by the police or the courts.

(15) A complaint can be submitted by any person who has knowledge of a court hearing involving a person whose name appears on the Council's register, who believes that the offences of which the practitioner has been found guilty call into question her future registration status.

How should a complaint alleging misconduct be made?

(16) Complaints alleging misconduct should be made in writing to the investigating officer of the National Board for Nursing, Midwifery and Health Visiting which is relevant to the home or work address of the practitioner concerned.

(17) The letter should set out the essential details of the complaint in succinct terms, and provide as much information as is available to assist identification of the practitioner on the Council's register.

What factors should a potential complainant bear in mind?

(18) The points made in paragraph 6 of this document are very important.

(19) If the case is referred to the Council by the relevant National Board for a Professional Conduct Committee hearing, evidence in support of the allegations of misconduct must be given by witnesses testifying under oath in a public hearing.

(20) Potential complaints must also note that the standards of evidence and proof required are the same as those applying in criminal courts. 'Hearsay' or 'indirect' evidence is not admissible. Before finding any allegation proved, the committee members, having heard evidence in accordance with strict rules, must be satisfied to the degree of being sure. Probability is not enough when the serious sanction of removing a person's right to practise is available to the committee.

What happens once a complaint alleging misconduct is made?

(21) The practitioner's name is identified on the Council's register and then an officer and solicitor for the relevant National Board will take action to assemble evidence available in support of the complaint.

(22) Guilt which has already been proven in a criminal court forms the basis on which the case will proceed. Further investigation is not required to establish the facts.

(23) In either case the practitioner is asked for a written statement, explanation or comment.

(24) The Investigating Committee of the relevant National Board then considers all the assembled information. It decides whether or not to refer the case to the Council's Professional Conduct Committee for a hearing with a view to removal from the register for misconduct. If it takes the view that the matters complained of are indicative of illness, the case can be referred for consideration by the Health Committee.

What special points apply to the Professional Conduct Committee when it considers a case?

(25) The points made in paragraph 6 of this document again apply.

(26) The purpose of the hearing is to concentrate on the matters which feature in the charges formally notified to the practitioner and is not to elicit evidence of other unsatisfactory behaviour.

(27) It is essential that the incident, if proved to the required standard, is considered in the context of its occurrence rather than in isolation.

(28) Information about the previous history of the respondent practitioner is extremely important. It sometimes emerges that the incident in question occurred when the pressure of work was severe, that the practitioner was immediately honest and open about it and that the previous record over many years was examplary.

(29) If, during the course of a hearing, evidence of possible ill health of the practitioner becomes available, the Professional Conduct Committee can decide to refer a case for consideration by the Health Committee.

What types of offence lead to removal from the register?

(30) The Council's Annual Reports from 1984 to 1989 provide information about how often particular types of proven charge have featured in cases which resulted in removal from the professional register.

(31) Practice related offences are always at or near the top of the list. These are offences which show a failure to honour the primacy of the interests of patients.

(32) Frequently occurring reasons for removal from the register are:

- Reckless and wilfully unskilful practice;
- Concealing untoward incidents;
- Failure to keep essential records;
- Falsifying records;
- Failure to protect or promote the interests of patients/clients;
- Failure to act knowing that a colleague or subordinate is improperly treating or abusing patients;
- Physical or verbal abuse of patients/clients;
- Abuse of patients by improperly withholding prescribed drugs, or administering unprescribed drugs or an excess of prescribed drugs;
- Theft from patients or employers;
- Drug related offences;
- Sexual abuse of patients;
- Breach of confidentiality.

(33) These categories of offence are not the only ones which have resulted in removal. They are simply those which have been regarded as particularly reprehensible. No two cases are the same in their details or context.

What types of case referred for Professional Conduct Committee hearings have not culminated in removal?

(34) Attention has already been drawn to the required standards of evidence and proof. Where that standard is not satisfied, the allegations are not proved and the respondent practitioner is declared not guilty of misconduct. A substantial number of cases to date have concluded in this way.

(35) There are a significant number of cases in which the facts are established, but which are not seen as misconduct by the Professional Conduct Committee when considered in context. This decision concludes the case.

(36) Cases most often found in this category include:

- Offences related to motor vehicles;
- Issues that relate specifically to employment, such as leaving duty early without authority, overtime claims in excess of hours worked, or mistakes disclosed by the practitioner which were made under pressure of work;
- Cases where the practitioner's failure was effectively a failure to achieve the impossible in the particular circumstances that applied;
- Cases which result from careful and conscientious exercise of professional

judgment by the practitioner and which can be justified as reasonable in the circumstances and at the time the decision was taken;
- Situations where the case has been brought by a complainant measuring the actions of the practitioner against outdated practices and norms.

(37) When the facts alleged and misconduct are proved, certain reasons may emerge which lead the Professional Conduct Committee to decide that the practitioner's name should not be removed from the Register. These have included cases where:

- The incident was isolated and uncharacteristic and the practitioner appears to have learnt lessons from it;
- There were, at the time, overwhelming personal problems which led the practitioner to behave inappropriately and which have since been resolved;
- The practitioner has been retained in employment and is the subject of good reports;
- The practitioner, having been responsible for an error, has made no attempt to conceal it and has immediately reported it in the interests of the patient;
- With hindsight it is clear that the incident was an error in professional judgment rather than a culpable act;
- The practitioner was one of a number involved, but the only person to be the subject of the complaint;
- Removal is judged to be too harsh a response to the facts that have been established.

(38) In addition to the above, there have been rare occasions where the incident or incidents have occurred in a stressful work setting with highly dependent patients, poor staffing and limited support resources. Senior professional managers appear to have been fully aware of the deficiencies of the work environment but have taken no effective remedial action. In these circumstances, and in those particular cases heard by the Professional Conduct Committee, it was believed that removal of the name of the practitioner would be an inappropriate response to the problem.

COMPLAINTS ALLEGING UNFITNESS TO PRACTISE DUE TO ILLNESS

Who can express concern that a practitioner may be unfit to practise due to illness?

(39) As with misconduct, anyone can express concern and initiate the process through which a practitioner's possible unfitness due to illness will be assessed and a decision made about her registration status. Such an expression of concern should be made direct to the Council.

(40) An Investigating Committee or Professional Conduct Committee can refer a case which has been brought to its attention as an allegation of misconduct.

When should concern that a practitioner's fitness to practise is impaired, be expressed to the Council?

(41) Where such concerns emerge in the course of Investigating Committee or Professional Conduct Committee consideration of a case, and become a matter of formal record, the case is transferred immediately for assembly of medical evidence.

(42) In all other cases, a person who becomes concerned about a practitioner's illness or disability should formally express this concern as soon as she is satisfied that it appears to have seriously impaired the ability to practise safely, provided the illness leading to impairment is not of a short-term nature. This action should not be seen as an alternative to offering local assistance to a practitioner who appears to be unwell.

How should concerns that a practitioner's fitness to practise is impaired by illness be brought to the attention of the Council?

(43) A letter which provides brief details of the known illness or symptomatic behaviour giving rise to concern, together with sufficient information to identify the practitioner, should be sent directly to the Council. This category of case is known as a direct referral.

(44) Letters should be addressed to:

Assistant Registrar, Professional Conduct
United Kingdom Central Council for Nursing,
Midwifery and Health Visiting
23 Portland Place
London
W1N 3AF

(45) Where possible, copies of any documents providing further information about the alleged unfitness to practise should be enclosed with the letter.

What happens next in a direct referral case?

(46) Using the letter and enclosures from the person making the referral, the Council's solicitor draws up a statutory declaration for that person to sign. This document is a requirement of the law; without it an investigation of a practitioner's alleged unfitness to practise cannot proceed.

(47) Once the statutory declation has been signed and returned to the Council, the case is formally opened and considered by a group of Council members (the Panel of Screeners) who look at documentary evidence and decide whether it should be pursued or closed. If it is to be pursued, the Screeners then decide on the category of specialist medical examiners to whom they wish the practitioner to be referred.

What happens next in a health case referred from an Investigating Committee or Professional Conduct Committee

(48) The decision that the practitioner's fitness to practise is a question in dispute has already been addressed by the referring committee. The role of the Screeners is limited to selecting the category of examiners. In exceptional cases, the Screeners may ask the Chairman of Council to use the personal authority conferred by the statutory rules and send a case back to the referring committee for further consideration.

By whom are the medical examinations conducted?

(49) The Council is required to maintain a panel of medical examiners covering a wide

range of specialities. These examiners are appointed after nomination by specialist bodies such as the Royal Colleges of Physicians and Psychiatrists.

(50) Whenever possible, practitioners are referred to examiners who are geographically convenient. The medical examiners, however, will never be persons who practise in the same area as the referred practitioner. The full cost of examinations and travel is met by the Council.

Do the Screeners consider the case again?

(51) In direct referral cases the original documents, now supplemented by the reports prepared by the medical examiners, are considered by the Screeners. They must decide whether to close the case or forward it to the Health Committee.

Does the practitioner have access to the medical reports?

(52) Yes. As soon as reports are received by Council's staff, they are copied and sent to the practitioner, who then has a period of time to decide whether to choose medical practitioners from whom to commission additional reports.

How is the Health Committee hearing conducted?

(53) Because of the nature of the material to be considered, the hearing is conducted in private. The Health Committee for each case is composed of five Council members supported by an officer and a legal assessor. One of the medical examiners, whose reports form an essential part of the material before the committee, must be present. The practitioner is encouraged to attend and may require that both examiners attend. She can be represented by a person or organisation of her choice and may also bring medical advisers and relatives or friends.

(54) In the majority of cases the practitioner accepts the general accuracy and conclusions of the medical reports and allows them, together with any other medical reports commissioned, to form the basis of discussion about the contention that fitness to practise may be seriously impaired by illness.

(55) On very rare occasions in direct referral cases, the practitioner refuses the invitation to medical examination by the Council's selected examiners and exercises the right to have the persons making the allegations, together with other witnesses to the behaviour on which the allegation is based, called to give evidence under oath. In such a case, one or more of the medical practitioners drawn from the Council's panel of examiners will attend in the role of medical assessor to advise the committee.

What types of illness have often culminated in removal from the register since the Health Committee commenced its work in 1984?

(56) Each case is the subject of detailed consideration and any illness that results in serious impairment of fitness to practise can result in removal.

(57) It is a matter of record that conditions which have featured most frequently where practitioners' names have been removed from the register have been alcohol dependence, other drug dependence and various forms of mental illness.

SUMMARY AND CONCLUSION

(58) This document should not be read as an attempt to deter potential complainants

from seeking investigation and judgment of those actions or omissions of practition-ers which cause them particular concern, nor should it be read as an attempt to deter the reporting of ill practitioners in whose hands vulnerable patients and clients may be at risk. On the contrary, by providing information about the system, the standards that must be satisfied and the outcome of cases in the recent past it seeks to make sure that there is no delay to cases which need to be dealt with expeditiously in the interests of patients and clients.

(59) It has been stated that complaints should be made, '. . . with a view to removal from the register. . .'. If this is not the outcome which the potential complainant is seeking, she should think carefully and consider seeking advice before submitting the complaint.

(60) This document has been prepared to help you understand the process by which the statutory bodies, created by the Nurses, Midwives and Health Visitors Act 1979, deal with allegations of misconduct and with complaints alleging unfitness to practise due to illness.

(61) In particular, it seeks to assist those who may be considering making complaints about persons whose names are on the Council's register.

(62) Persons considering forwarding complaints alleging misconduct should ask them-selves whether they personally consider the matter to be misconduct in a professional sense before formally making a complaint against a named individual.

(63) It is wise to refer to the two items the Professional Conduct Committee members will have in mind. The first of these is the definition of misconduct in the statutory rules which states that 'Misconduct is conduct unworthy of a nurse, midwife or health visitor.' The second is the Code of Professional Conduct for the Nurse, Midwife and Health Visitor, a copy of which is available from the distribution office of the Council.

(64) If the potential complainant takes the view that the matter (if proved to the required standard) is misconduct, she ought to go further and consider whether it raises a question only about the practitioner's appropriateness to continue in her present post, or, alternatively, raises serious questions about her appropriateness to practise with patients/clients. If the conclusion is that it falls into the latter category, it should be forwarded. If it is the former, there may be little point in forwarding the complaint. Only the potential complainant can make this decision.

(65) If the potential complainant takes the view that a particular practitioner is ill, she needs to consider carefully whether the illness seriously impairs the practitioner's fitness to practise.

(66) Questions arising from this advisory document should be directed to the Assistant Registrar, Professional Conduct, at the Council.

November 1990

Annexe A

**A simplified illustration of the process by which
an allegation of misconduct is considered**

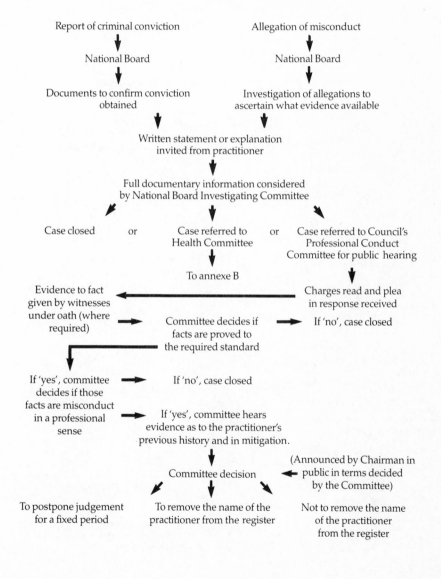

Annexe B

**A simplified illustration of the process by which
complaints alleging unfitness to practise are considered**

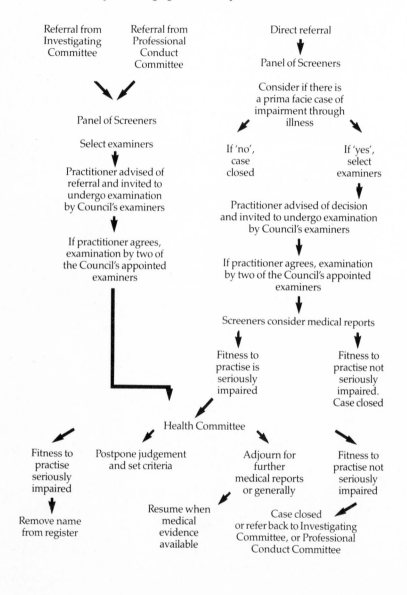

Appendix 2

Exercising accountability

A. INTRODUCTION

(1) The United Kingdom Central Council for Nursing, Midwifery and Health Visiting regulates the nursing, midwifery and health visiting professions in the public interest.

The UKCC was established by the Nurses, Midwives and Health Visitors Act 1979.

Section 2(1) of the Nurses, Midwives and Health Visitors Act 1979 states that 'The *principal functions of the Central Council shall be to establish and improve standards of training and professional conduct'.*

Section 2(5) of the same Act moves from the requirement to improve conduct to one of the methods to be employed when it states that 'The *powers of the Council shall include that of providing in such manner as it thinks fit, advice for nurses, midwives and health visitors on standards of professional conduct'.*

(2) The Code of Professional Conduct for the Nurse, Midwife and Health Visitor is the Council's definitive advice on professional conduct to its practitioners. In this extremely important document practitioners on the UKCC's register find a clear and unequivocal statement as to what their regulatory body expects of them. It therefore also provides the backcloth against which any alleged misconduct on their part will be judged.

The Code of Professional Conduct is considered to be

a statement to the profession of the primacy of the interests of the patient or client.

a statement of the profession's values.

a portrait of the practitioner which the Council believes to be needed and which the Council wishes to see within the profession.

(3) The Council has already published three advisory documents to supplement the Code of Professional Conduct. Practitioners now seek:

(i)   elaboration of clauses 10 & 11 of the Code and support for their position when doing as these clauses require. These Clauses state that:

'Each *registered nurse, midwife and health visitor is accountable for his or her practice and, in the exercise of professional accountability, shall:*

10. *Have regard to the environment of care and its physical, psychological and social effects on patients/clients, and also to the adequacy of resources, and make known to appropriate persons or authorities any circumstances which could place patients/clients in jeopardy or which militate against safe standards of practice.*

147

11. *Have regard to the workload of and the pressures on professional colleagues and subordinates and take appropriate action if these are seen to be such as to constitute abuse of the individual practitioner and/or to jeopardise safe standards of practice'.*

(ii) advice and guidance on issues related to consent and the general subject of truth telling.

(iii) advice and guidance on that part of the practitioner's role which concerns advocacy on behalf of patients and clients.

(iv) elaboration of clause 5 of the Code which states that each registered nurse, midwife and health visitor shall:

5. *'Work in a collaborative and co-operative manner with other health care professionals and recognise and respect their particular contributions within the health care team.'*

(v) advice and guidance on issues related to contentious treatments and conscientious objection.

This document provides a response to those requests, aims to assist professional practitioners to exercise their judgment and reinforces the importance of the Code of Professional Conduct.

B. THE CODE OF PROFESSIONAL CONDUCT AND THE SUBJECT OF ACCOUNTABILITY

(1) This new UKCC advisory document has been produced in order to establish more clearly the extent of accountability of registered nurses, midwives and health visitors and to assist them in the exercise of professional accountability in order to achieve high standards of professional practice.

(2) The Code begins with an unequivocal statement

'Each registered nurse, midwife and health visitor shall act, at all times, in such a manner as to justify public trust and confidence, to uphold and enhance the good standing and reputation of the profession, to serve the interests of society and above all to safeguard the interests of individual patients and clients'.

This introductory clause indicates that a registered practitioner is accountable for her actions as a professional at all times, whether engaged in current practice or not and whether on or off duty.

In situations where the practitioner is employed she will be accountable to the employer for providing a service which she is employed to provide and for the proper use of the resources made available by the employer for this purpose.

In the circumstances described in the preceding two paragraphs the practitioner has an ultimate accountability to the UKCC for any failure to satisfy the requirements of the introductory paragraph of the Code of Professional Conduct.

The words 'accountable' and 'accountability' each occur only once in the Code, both being found in the stem paragraph out of which the subsequent 14 clauses grow. They do, however, provide its central focus as the Code is built upon the expectation that practitioners will conduct themselves in the manner it describes.

(3) Accountability is an integral part of professional practice, since, in the course of that

practice, the practitioner has to make judgments in a wide variety of circumstances and be answerable for those judgments. The Code of Professional Conduct does not seek to state all the circumstances in which accountability has to be exercised, but to state important principles.

The primacy of the interests of the public and patient or client provide the first theme of the Code and establish the point that, in determining his or her approach to professional practice, the individual nurse, midwife or health visitor should recognise that the interests of public and patient must predominate over those of practitioner and profession. The second major theme is the exercise by each practitioner of personal professional accountability in such a manner as to respect the primacy of those interests.

(4) The Code of Professional Conduct states unequivocally that all practitioners who are registered on the UKCC's register are required to seek to set and achieve high standards and thereby honour the requirement of *Clause 1 of the Code* which states that each registered nurse, midwife and health visitor shall:

1. *'Act always in such a way as to promote and safeguard the wellbeing and interests of patients and clients'.*

It is recognised that, in many situations in which practitioners practice, there may be a tension between the maintenance of standards and the availability or use of resources. It is essential, however, that the profession, both through its regulatory body (the UKCC) and its individual practitioners, adheres to its desire to enhance standards and to achieve high standards rather than to simply accept minimum standards. Practitioners must seek remedies in those situations where factors in the environment obstruct the achievement of high standards: to start from a compromise position and silently to tolerate poor standards is to act in a manner contrary to the interests of patients or clients, and thus renege on personal professional accountability.

C. CONCERN IN RESPECT OF THE ENVIRONMENT OF CARE

(1) The dilemma for practitioners in many settings in respect of the environment of care is very real and has been well documented. If practitioners express concern at the situations which obstruct the achievement of satisfactory standards they risk censure from their employers. On the other hand, failure to make concerns known renders practitioners vulnerable to complaint to their regulatory body (the UKCC) for failing to satisfy its standards and places their registration status in jeopardy.

The sections of the Code of Professional Conduct that are particularly relevant to this issue are the introductory paragraphs and clauses numbered 1, 2, 3, 10 & 11. *These parts of the Code apply to each and every person on the Council's register. Whether engaged in direct care of the patient or client, or further removed but in a position to exert influence over the setting in which that contact exists, the practitioner is subject to the Code and has accountability for her actions or omissions.*

(2) The import of the Sections of the Code referred to is that, having, as part of her professional accountability, the responsibility to *'serve the interests of society and above all to safeguard the interests of individual patients and clients'* and to *'act always in such a way as to promote and safeguard the wellbeing and interests of patients/clients'*, the registered nurse, midwife and health visitor must make appropriate representations about the environment of care:

(a) where patients or clients seem likely to be placed in jeopardy and/or standards of practice endangered;

(b) where the staff in such settings are at risk because of the pressure of work and/or inadequacy of resources (which again places patients at risk); and

(c) where valuable resources are being used inappropriately.

This is an essential part of the communication process that should operate in any facility providing health care, to ensure that those who determine, manage and allocate resources do so with full knowledge of the consequences for the achievement of satisfactory standards. Nurses, midwives and health visitors in management positions should ensure that all relevant information on standards of practice is obtained and communicated with others involved in health policy and management in the interests of standards and safety.

(3) Practitioners engaged in direct patient or client care should not be deterred from making representations of their concerns regarding the environment of care simply because they believe that resources are unavailable or that action will not result. The immediate professional manager to whom such information is given, having assessed that information, should ensure that it is communicated to more senior professional managers. This is important in order that, should complaints be made about the practitioners involved in delivering care, the immediate and senior managers will be able to confirm that the perceived inadequacies in the environment of care have been drawn to their attention.

It is clearly wrong for any practitioner to pretend to be coping with the workload, to delude herself into the conviction that things are better than they really are, to aid and abet the abuse and breakdown of a colleague, or to tolerate in silence any matters in her work setting that place patients at risk, jeopardise standards of practice, or deny patients privacy and dignity.

In summary, Section C of this document simply restates the UKCC's expectations (set out in the Code of Professional Conduct) that while accepting their responsibilities and doing their best to fulfil them, practitioners on its register will ensure that the reality of their clinical environment and practice is made known to and understood by appropriate persons or authorities, doing this as an expression of their personal professional accountability exercised in the public interest. An essential part of this process is the making of contemporaneous and accurate records of the consequences for patients and clients if they have not been given the care they required.

(4) *The Code of Professional Conduct applies to all persons on the Council's register irrespective of the post held. Their perspective will vary with their role, but they share the overall responsibility for care. No practitioner will find support in the Code or from the UKCC for the contention that genuinely held concerns should not be expressed or, if expressed, should attract censure.*

D. CONSENT AND TRUTH

(1) It is self-evident that for it to have any meaning consent has to be informed. For the purposes of this document 'informed consent' means that the practitioner involved explains the intended test or procedure to the patient without bias and in as much detail (including detail of possible reactions, complications, side effects and social or personal ramifications) as the patient requires. In the case of an unquestioning patient the practitioner assesses and determines what information the patient needs so that the patient may make an informed decisions. The practitioner should impart the information in a sensitive manner, recognising that it might cause distress. The patient must be given time to consider the information before being required to give the consent unless it is an emergency situation

(2) In many instances the practitioner involved in obtaining informed consent would be a registered medical practitioner. In those circumstances it is the medical practitioner who should impart the information and subsequently seek the signed consent. Normally, in respect of patients in hospital, there are good reasons why the information should be given and the consent sought in the presence of a nurse, midwife or health visitor. Where the procedure or test is to be performed by a nurse, midwife or health visitor the standards described in the preceding paragraph apply to the consent sought.

(3) If the nurse, midwife or health visitor does not feel that sufficient information has been given in terms readily understandable to the patient so as to enable him to make a truly informed decision, it is for her to state this opinion and seek to have the situation remedied. The practitioner might decide not to co-operate with a procedure if convinced that the decision to agree to it being performed was not truly informed. Discussion of such matters between the health professionals concerned should not take place in the presence of patients.

In certain situations and with certain client groups the practitioner's level of responsibility in this respect is greatly increased where she stands in 'loco parentis' for a patient or client.

(4) There are occasions on which, although the patient has been given information by the medical practitioner about an intended procedure for which he has given consent, his subsequent statements and questions to a nurse, midwife or health visitor indicate a failure to understand what is to be done, its risks and its ramifications. Where this proves to be the case it is necessary for that practitioner, in the patient's interest, to recall the relevant medical practitioner so that the deficiencies can be remedied without delay.

The purpose of this approach is to ensure that all professional practitioners involved in the patient's care respect the primacy of that patient's interests, honour their personal professional accountability and avoid the risk of complaint or charges of assault. The practitioner who properly fulfils her responsibilities in this respect should be recognised by medical colleagues as a source of support and information to improve the overall care of the patient.

(5) The concept of informed consent and that of truth telling are closely related. If it is to be believed that, on occasions, practitioners withhold information from their patients the damage to public trust and confidence in the profession, on which the introduction to the Code of Professional Conduct places great emphasis, will be enormous.

(6) This is yet another area in which judgments have to be made and introduces another facet of the exercise of accountability. If it is accepted that the patient has a right to information about his condition it follows that the professional practitioners involved in his care have a duty to provide such information. Recognition of the patient's condition and the likely effect of the information might lead the professionals to be selective about 'what' and 'when' but the responsibility is on them to provide information. There may be occasions on which, after consultation with the relatives of a patient by the health professionals involved in that patient's care, some information is temporarily withheld. If, however, something less than the whole truth is told at a particular point in time it should never be because the practitioner is unable to cope with the effects of telling the whole truth. Such controlled release of information (i.e. less than the whole truth) should only ever be in the interests of the patient, and the practitioner should be able to justify the action taken.

(7) It is recognised that this is an area in which there is the potential for conflict between professionals involved in the care of the same patient or client. The existence of good, trusting relationships between professionals concerned will promote the development of agreed approaches to truth telling. This subject should be discussed between all the

professional practitioners involved so that the rights of patients are not affected adversely. This should minimise the number of occasions on which, after a patient or client has been given incomplete information, a nurse, midwife or health visitor is faced with a request for the whole truth. Accountability can never be exercised by ignoring the rights and interests of the patient or client.

E. ADVOCACY ON BEHALF OF PATIENTS AND CLIENTS

(1) The introductory paragraphs of the Code of Professional Conduct, together with several of its clauses, indicate clearly the expectation that the practitioner will accept a role as an advocate on behalf of his or her patients/clients. Opinions vary as to what exactly that means. Some tend to want to identify advocacy as a separate and distinct subject. It is not. It is a component of many professional activities of this and other professions. Some of these professional activities are the subject of other sections of this document.

(2) *Advocacy is concerned with promoting and safeguarding the wellbeing and interests of patients and clients. It is not concerned with conflict for its own sake.* It is important that this fact is recognised, since some practitioners seem to regard advocacy on behalf of patients or clients as an adversarial activity and feel either attracted to it or not able to accept it for that reason. Dictionaries define an advocate as 'one who pleads the cause of another' or 'one who recommends or urges something' and indicates that advocacy is a positive, constructive activity.

(3) There are occasions on which the practitioner's advocacy role has to be exercised to 'plead the cause of another' where, in the case of any person incapable of making informed decisions, the parents or relatives withhold consent for treatment which the various practitioners involved believe to be in the best interests of the patient. The parents or relatives, from their knowledge of the patient, will also have an opinion as to what constitutes his or her best interests. There have been a limited number of cases in which the courts have taken the view that the parents or relatives have not decided in the patient's best interests. Taking the right of decision away from the parents or relatives should only occur in the rarest of cases. The practitioner's advocacy role in situations of this kind requires knowledge of the patient's condition and prognosis, sensitivity to the feelings of the parents or relatives and considerable empathy.

(4) *To fulfil the Council's expectations set out in the Code is, therefore, to be the advocate for the patient or client in this sense. Each practitioner must determine exactly how this aspect of personal professional accountability is satisfied within her particular sphere of practice. This requires the exercise of judgment as to the 'when' and 'how'. The practitioner must be sure that it is the interests of the patient or client that are being promoted rather than the patient or client being used as a vehicle for the promotion of personal or sectional professional interests. The Code of Professional Conduct envisages the role of patient or client advocate as an integral and essential aspect of good professional practice.'*

(5) Just as the practice of nursing involves the practitioner in assisting the patient with those physical activities which he would do for himself were be able, so too the exercise of professional accountability involves the practitioner in assisting the patient by making such representations on his behalf as he would make himself if he were able.

F. COLLABORATION AND CO-OPERATION IN CARE

(1) Clause 5 of the Code of Professional Conduct requires that *'Each registered nurse, midwife and health visitor, in the exercise of professional accountability shall work in a collaborative and co-operative manner with other health care professionals and*

recognise and respect their particular contributions within the health care team'. This clause deliberately emphasises the importance of collaboration and co-operation and, by implication, the importance of the avoidance of dispute and the promotion of good relationships and a spirit of co-operation and mutual respect within the team.

(2) It does so because it is clearly impossible for any one profession or agency to possess all the knowledge, skill and resources to be employed in meeting the total health care needs of society. The delivery of full and appropriate care to patients/clients frequently necessitates the participation of professional practitioners from more than one profession, their efforts often being supplemented by other agencies and persons.

The UKCC recognises the complexity of medical and health care and stresses the need to appreciate the complementary contribution of the professions and others involved.

The delivery of care is therefore often a multi-profession and multi-agency activity which, in order to be effective, must be based on mutual understanding, trust, respect and co-operation.

(3) It is self-evident that collaborative and co-operative working is essential if patients and clients are to be provided with the care they need and if it is to be of the quality required. It is worthy of note that this concept of teamwork is evident in many situations in which the care of patients and clients is a shared responsibility. Unfortunately there are exceptions. Experience has demonstrated that such co-operation and collaboration is not always easily achieved if:

(a) individual members of the team have their own specific and separate objectives; or
(b) one member of the team seeks to adopt a dominant role to the exclusion of the opinions, knowledge and skill of its other members.

In such circumstances it is important to stress that the interests of the patient or client must remain paramount.

(4) The UKCC and the General Medical Council agree that there is a range of issues which calls for co-operation between the professions at both national and local level and wish to encourage this co-operation.

(5) In spite of acceptance of the importance of co-operation and collaboration, differences can sometimes occur within the team regarding appropriate care and treatment. Such conflict can become an influence for good if it results in full discussion between members of the team. It may prove harmful to the care and treatment of patients or clients unless resolved in a manner which recognises the special contribution of each professional group, agency and individual and ensures that the interests and needs of the patient or client remain paramount.

(6) *Collaboration and co-operation between health care professionals is also necessary in both research and planning related to the provision or improvement of services.* This may sometimes give rise to concern where one professional group is requested to pass information (obtained by its members in the course of professional practice) to a member of another professional group to use for a purpose other than that for which it was obtained and recorded. That level of concern will inevitably rise unless it can be seen that the purpose for which the information is required is valid, the information is made available only to persons bound by the same standards of confidentiality and the means of storage of that information is secure.

This should not present a problem where consent can be obtained from the patients or clients to whom the information relates or from relatives who have been provided with the relevant information. In certain fields, such as care of the elderly and persons with mental illness and mental handicap, the information gathering and research geared to the provision of services for these client groups may need to proceed without specific consent. This should only occur where the individuals receiving care are unable to give informed consent and where there is no close contact with relatives. Those who proceed without consent in these particular circumstances must be satisfied that their activities will not affect the current provision of care adversely and that the activity is directed to the provision of appropriate or improved services for future recipients of care.

It is anticipated that disputes will be avoided by relevant inter-professional discussions in advance of submission of the projects for approval by the appropriate ethical committees. Where a dispute does arise it should be resolved between colleagues and the ethical committee.

Clause 9 of the Code of Professional Conduct and the UKCC's Advisory Paper on 'Confidentiality' provide further sources of reference for nurses, midwives and health visitors in respect of this aspect of practice.

G. OBJECTION TO PARTICIPATION IN CARE AND TREATMENT

(1) *Clause 7 of the Code of Professional Conduct states:*

'Make known to an appropriate person or authority any conscientious objection which may be relevant to professional practice'.

(2) The law does not provide a general opportunity for practitioners to register a conscientious objection to participation in care and treatment. That right applies in respect of termination of pregnancy only (not the care of the patient thereafter) under the terms of Section 4 of the Abortion Act 1967.

(3) Some practitioners choose not to participate in certain other forms of treatment on the grounds of conscience. Since the law provides no basic right to such a refusal it is imperative that any practitioner should be careful not to accept employment in a post where it is known that a form of treatment to which she has a conscientious objection is regularly used. In circumstances where a practitioner finds that a form of treatment to which she objects, but which is not usually employed, is to be used she must declare that objection with sufficient time for her managers to make alternative staffing arrangements and must not refuse to participate in emergency treatment.

Some practitioners may object to participation in certain forms of treatment, such as resuscitative treatment of the elderly, the transfusion of blood, or electro-convulsive therapy. These practitioners must respect clause 7 of the Code and make their position clear to their professional colleagues and managers, and recognise that this may have implications for their contract of employment.

(4) Objection to participation in treatment does not only occur as a product of conscience. It is the Council's stated position that, on each and every occasion a prescribed medication is being administered, the practitioner should ensure that, in her view, the patient is not presenting symptoms that contra-indicate its administration. The practitioner who is concerned about the administration of a particular drug in these circumstances might reasonably ask the prescribing doctor to attend the patient and, if the prescriber still requires it to be given, to request her to administer the medication if not fully reassured. The practitioner involved in such an incident should make a detailed record of the reasons why she felt concern and, if so, why she declined to administer prescribed medication.

(5) The principle that applies in the previous paragraph can also be applied in appropriate

circumstances to substances that are prescribed for topical use including wound dressings. Where the practitioner attending the patient believes (from knowledge, published research evidence or from previous experience) that the prescribed substance may be harmful, or even more so where it is evident that it is actively harmful, she should make a record of the condition of the wound or site (where appropriate including a photographic record) and ask the prescribing medical practitioner to attend.

If the prescription stands after medical examination the practitioner, having chosen either to respond to the prescription or not, should make a detailed record of the reasons for her expressed concern and subsequent actions.

It is believed that the spirit of co-operation and mutual respect referred to at paragrph F1 of this document should make such situations exceptional.

(6) Objections to participation in treatment are not always associated with the nature or form of treatment or its appropriateness in a particular set of circumstances. Some practitioners indicate their wish or active intention to refuse to participate in the delivery of care to patients with certain conditions. Such refusal may be associated particularly with patients suffering from Hepatitis B Infection and those with Acquired Immune Deficiency Syndrome, AIDS Related Complex or who are HIV sero-positive but asymptomatic.

Those who seek the UKCC's support for such actual or intended refusal are informed that the Code of Professional Conduct does not provide a formula for being selective about the categories of patient or client for whom the practitioner will care. To seek to be so selective is to demonstrate unacceptable conduct. The UKCC expects its practitioners to adopt a non-judgmental approach in the exercise of their caring role.

H. SUMMARY OF THE PRINCIPLES AGAINST WHICH TO EXERCISE ACCOUNTABILITY

(1) The interests of the patients or client are paramount.

(2) Professional accountability must be exercised in such a manner as to ensure that the primacy of the interests of patients or clients is respected and must not be overidden by those of the professions or their practitioners.

(3) The exercise of accountability requires the practitioner to seek to achieve and maintain high standards.

(4) Advocacy on behalf of patients or clients is an essential feature of the exercise of accountability by a professional practitioner.

(5) The role of other persons in the delivery of health care to patients or clients must be recognised and respected, provided that the first principle above is honoured.

(6) Public trust and confidence in the profession is dependent on its practitioners being seen to exercise their accountability responsibly.

(7) Each registered nurse, midwife or health visitor must be able to justify any action or decision not to act taken in the course of her professional practice.

Appendix 3

Confidentiality

A. INTRODUCTION

(1) *The Code of Professional Conduct for the Nurse, Midwife and Health Visitor (Second Edition) published by the United Kingdom Central Council for Nursing, Midwifery and Health Visiting is:*

a statement to the profession of the primacy of the interests of the patient or client;

one of the principal means by which the Council is seeking to comply with Section 2(5) of the Nurses, Midwives and Health Visitors Act 1979 and give advice to its practitioners on standards of professional conduct;

a portrait of the practitioner the Council believes to be needed and wishes to see within the profession.

(2) In approving the terms of this edition of the *Code* the Council authorised the publication of key statements on a number of important professional issues.
(3) One of these key statements (Clause 9) concerns 'Confidentiality'. It reads:

'Each registered nurse, midwife and health visitor is accountable for his or her practice, and, in the exercise of professional accountability shall:

Respect confidential information obtained in the course of professional practice and refrain from disclosing such information without the consent of the patient/client, or a person entitled to act on his/her behalf, except where disclosure is required by law or by the order of a court or is necessary in the public interest.'

(4) It can be seen from the general description of the Code of Professional Conduct and the particular contents of Clause 9 that *breaches of confidentiality should be regarded as exceptional,* only occurring after careful consideration and the exercise of personal professional judgment.
(5) Any codified statements of this nature need continuous exploration, and on occasions a more detailed and authoritative elaboration. It is for the whole profession to recognise its responsibility to share in such exploration, to use the respective knowledge and skill of practitioners to facilitate it and to recognise the important contribution the professional press makes to this essential debate. The subject of confidentiality has emerged as one on which the profession's practitioners need the relevant clause in the Code of Professional Conduct to be developed more fully by the UKCC. It must be said, however, that *no exploration or elaboration by others alters the fact that the ultimate decision is that of the individual practitioner in the situation.*

The demand for elaboration of Clause 9 of the Code has focused particularly on *determining the difficult boundary that applies in any case between the expectations of patients/clients that information, whether recorded or not, obtained in the course of professional practice will not be disclosed, and the expectations of the public that they will not be put at risk because practitioners unreasonably withhold information.*

It is not the purpose of this document to seek to provide answers to the many dilemmas which practitioners face. It is necessary, however, to provide examples of them since they have been a backcloth against which the discussions culminating in the publication of this document have taken place.

Correspondence on this point has come (for example) from:

a sister in a psychiatric day hospital who found a patient possessed of large quantities of controlled drugs that he cannot have obtained legally;

a medical practitioner concerned that a community midwife reported to her employers the fact that while visiting the wife of a hospital employee in a professional capacity she saw substantial quantities of stolen hospital property;

a health visitor who has been told by one child that another child is being sexually abused;

Accident and Emergency Department nursing staff who found that the unconscious patient they were treating had a gun on his person;

nurses working in the community who had been instructed by their managers (following approval by an ethical committee) to give researchers direct access to confidential information in respect of patients, but who knew that the consent of those patients had not been sought;

psychiatric nurses who fear that information revealed by a patient in a therapeutic group may be passed on by other patients and that the nurses will be held responsible;

occupational health nurses faced with requests from their managers for information about employees;

community psychiatric nurses who were reluctant to comply with the instruction to put full names and addresses of patients visited on their travel expense claims;

a health visitor who had become aware that information she shared with a social worker in a case conference had been given in evidence in a Magistrates' Court;

practitioners who have chosen not to make a record of information given to them by patients in confidence, and who have later been worried about the propriety of their decision; and

a health authority chairman who asks 'Who is to define the public interest?' and 'How is the nurse to recognise the authenticity of the claim of public interest?'

The Council has been left in no doubt that it has a responsibility to address this important subject in greater depth.

As already stated, *the UKCC is not seeking to provide responses to those dilemmas since a judgment must be made by the individual practitioner concerned. It is instead seeking to provide guidance on disclosure of information*:

(a) to assist development of understanding about the nature and scope of the dilemma which practitioners face, and to encourage those who employ nurses, midwives and health visitors to recognise the difficult and stressful situations encountered by practitioners and to offer support and guidance, stimulate the discussion and develop and publicise policies on this important matter;
(b) to state certain principles which it is hoped will assist practitioners to consider situations which they encounter and to make sound professional judgments;
(c) to emphasise that the responsibility of whether or not information should be withheld or disclosed without the consent of the patient/client lies with the practitioner involved at the appropriate time and cannot be delegated;
(d) to stress that those who employ or supervise nurses, midwives and health visitors have an obligation to support these practitioners in discharging their responsibilities in respect of the right to disclose or withhold information using their professional judgment;
(e) to indicate the conditions which should be met before disclosure of information, so that the decision to either disclose or withhold information can be justified.

B. DEFINING TERMS

(1) What do we mean when we speak of something being 'Confidential'? Turn to almost any Dictionary and you find that the focal word in the definitions of 'confide', 'confidence' or 'confidential' is *'TRUST'*. To trust another person with private and personal information about yourself is a significant matter. *Where the person to whom that information is given is a nurse, midwife or health visitor the patient/client has a right to believe that this information, given in confidence in the expectation that it will be used only for the purposes for which it was given, will not be released to others without the consent of the patient/client.* The death of a patient/client does not absolve the practitioner from this obligation.

(2) Clearly it is impractical to obtain the consent of the patient/client every time that health care information needs to be shared with other health professionals, or other staff involved in the health care of that patient/client. Consent in these instances can be implied provided that it is known and understood by the patients/clients that such information needs to be made available to others involved in the delivery of his/her care. Patients/clients have a right to know the standards of confidentiality maintained by those providing their care, and these standards should be made known by the health professional at the first point of contact. These standards of confidentiality can be reinforced by the additional use of leaflets and posters where the health care is being delivered.

(3) When an individual practitioner considers that it is necessary to obtain the explicit consent of a patient/client before disclosing specific information, it is the responsibility of the practitioner to ensure that the patient/client can make as informed a response as possible as to whether that information can be disclosed or withheld.

(4) It is essential that nurses, midwives and health visitors recognise the fundamental right of their patients or clients to information about them being kept private and secure. This point is sharply reinforced by only brief consideration of the personal, social or legal repercussions which might follow unauthorised disclosure of information concerning a person's health or illness.

(5) *Disclosure of information occurs in the following ways:*

(a) with the consent of the patient/client;
(b) without the consent of the patient/client when the disclosure is required by law or order of a court;
(c) by accident;
(d) without the consent of the patient/client when the disclosure is considered necessary in the public interest.

It is the latter two categories that this Advisory Paper is particularly addressing, for a breach of confidentiality occurs if anyone deliberately or by accident gives information, which has been obtained in the course of professional practice, to a third party without the consent of the patient/client.

(6) The public interest, in the context of this Advisory Paper, is taken to mean the interests of an individual, of groups of individuals or society as a whole, and would (for example) encompass matter such as serious crime, child abuse and drug trafficking.

C. OWNERSHIP AND CARE OF CONFIDENTIAL INFORMATION

(1) The organisations which employ professional practitioner staff who make records (whether in the National Health Service or in other spheres of practice) are the legal owner of such records, but such ownership does not give them any legal right of access to the information contained in those records. The patient also is involved in the ownership. The ownership of a record is therefore irrelevant to the patient's right of confidentiality and his/her expectation that identifiable personal health information will not be disclosed without consent.

(2) In many situations genuine difficulties can be experienced in preventing the leakage of confidential information or its inadvertent spread into management layers leading to possible misuse. There is need for particular caution where a system of shared records is employed, it being incumbent on the author of any particular entry to satisfy himself or herself that other people with access to that shared record will respect the confidentiality of the information and will place neither the patient/client nor the author of the entry at risk by its release without consent.

(3) The task with which individual professional practitioners are faced is not limited to that of exercising a judgment as to what information can be or should be disclosed. It also includes that of ensuring or helping to ensure that record keeping systems are not such as to make the release of information possible or likely. Neither technology nor management convenience should be allowed to determine principles. Each practitioner has a responsibility to recognise that risks exist, and to satisfy himself or herself in respect of the system for storage and movement of records operated in the health care setting in which he or she works and to ensure that it is secure. The concern for the environment of care for which each practitioner is held accountable under the terms of clause 10 of the Code of Professional Conduct for the Nurse, Midwife and Health Visitor extends to include this.

(4) The practitioner should act so as to ensure that he/she does not become a channel through which confidential information obtained in the course of professional practice is inadvertently released. The dangerous consequences of careless talk in public places cannot be overstated.

(5) Where access to the records of patients or clients is necessary so that students may be assisted to achieve the necessary knowledge and competence it must be recognised that the same principles of confidentiality stated earlier in this document extend to them and their teachers. The same applies to those engaged in research. It is incumbent on the

practitioner(s) responsible for the security of the information contained in these records to ensure that access to it is closely supervised, and occurs within the context of the teacher and student undertaking to respect its confidentiality, and in knowledge of the fact that the teacher has accepted responsibility to ensure that students understand the requirement for confidentiality and the need to observe local policies for the handling and storage of records. It is expected that the student or teacher who is active in giving care as a practitioner will apprise the patient of their role, thus enabling the patient who is so capable to control the information flow. Where deemed necessary the recipient of confidential information from a patient/client will advise him/her that the information will be conveyed to the nurse, midwife or health visitor involved in his/her care on a continuing basis.

(6) It is advisable that the contracts of employment of all employees not directly involved with patients/clients but who have access to or handle confidential records contain clauses which emphasise the principles of confidentiality and state the disciplinary consequences of breaching them. Paragraph 3.20 of the Report from the Confidentiality Working Group of the DHSS Steering Group on Health Services Information suggests a form of words worthy of consideration as follows:

'In the course of your duties you may have access to confidential material about patients, members of staff or other health service business. On no account must information relating to identifiable patients be divulged to anyone other than authorised persons, for example medical, nursing or other professional staff, as appropriate, who are concerned directly with the care, diagnosis and/or treatment of the patient. If you are in any doubt whatsoever as to the authority of a person or body asking for information of this nature you must seek advice from your superior officer. Similarly, no information of a personal or confidential nature concerning individual members of staff should be divulged to anyone without the proper authority having first been given. Failure to observe these rules will be regarded by your employers as serious misconduct which could result in serious disciplinary action being taken against you, including dismissal.'

The circumstances in which a nurse, midwife or health visitor chooses to disclose or withhold confidential information are explored in Section D.

D. DELIBERATE BREACH OF CONFIDENTIALITY IN THE PUBLIC INTEREST OR THAT OF THE INDIVIDUAL PATIENT/CLIENT

(1) The examples given in paragraph A5 remind us that we live in a real world, and that sometimes there are a range of interests to consider.

Pressure is often exerted on practitioners to breach the principle of keeping confidential and maintaining the security of information elicited from patients/clients in the privileged circumstances of a professional relationship. This should not be regarded as surprising, since 'Confidentiality' is a rule with certain exceptions. There is no statutory right of confidentiality; but there is also no bar to an aggrieved individual bringing a common law case before a civil court alleging breach of confidentiality and seeking financial recompense.

It is essential that before determining that a particular set of circumstances constitute such an exception, the practitioner must be satisfied that the best interests of the patient/

client are served thereby or the wider public interest necessitates disclosure.

(2) The needs of the community can, on occasions, take precedence over the individual's rights as for example in those situations where a Court rules that the administration of justice demands that a professional confidence be broken or the law requires that patient confidence be breached.

(3) In many other situations sharing of confidential information occurs by intention. This is the case where information obtained in the course of professional practice is shared with other professionals in the health and social work fields in the belief that to do so is in the interests of the patient/client. Legislation concerned with data protection and its associated codes is not intended to prevent the exchange of information between professional staff who share the care of the patient/client. It is, however, the duty of the practitioner who obtains and holds the information to ensure, as far as is reasonable, before its release that it is being imparted in strict professional confidence and for a specific purpose. The same duty applies where the practitioner is contributing to a shared record. Wherever possible the consent of the patient/client to the sharing of information should first be obtained.

(4) The situations that are the most exceptional and problematic for the practitioner are those where the deliberate decision to withhold confidential information or disclose it to a third party can have very serious consequences. The information can have been given to the practitioner in the strictest confidence or the practitioner may have obtained the information inadvertently in the course of his or her professional practice. The decision as to whether to make a record of such information, like the decision as to whether or not to disclose, poses many dilemmas, for the situations are invariably complex. In some instances the practitioner can be under pressure to divulge information but it must be emphasised that the responsibility lies with him or her as an individual. This responsibility cannot be delegated.

(5) In all cases where the practitioner deliberately discloses or withholds information in what he/she believes the public interest he/she must be able to justify the decision. These situations can be particularly stressful, especially where vulnerable groups are concerned, as disclosure may mean the involvement of a third party as in the case of children or the mentally handicapped. *Practitioners should always take the opportunity to discuss the matter fully with other practitioners* (not only or necessarily fellow nurses, midwives and health visitors), and if appropriate consult with a professional organisation before making a decision. There will often be ramifications and these are best explored before a final decision as to whether to withhold or disclose information is made.

Once having made a decision the practitioner should write down the reasons either in the appropriate record or in a special note that can be kept on file. The practitioner can then justify the action taken should that subsequently become necessary, and can also at a later date review the decision in the light of future developments.

E. SUMMARY OF THE PRINCIPLES ON WHICH TO BASE PROFESSIONAL JUDGMENT IN MATTERS OF CONFIDENTIALITY

(1) That a patient/client has a right to expect that information given in confidence will be used only for the purpose for which it was given and will not be released to others without their consent.

(2) That practitioners recognise the fundamental right of their patients/clients to have information about them held in secure and private storage.

(3) That, where it is deemed appropriate to share information obtained in the course of

professional practice with other health or social work practitioners, the practitioner who obtained the information must ensure, as far as is reasonable, before its release that it is being imparted in strict professional confidence and for a specific purpose.

(4) That the responsibility to either disclose or withhold confidential information in the public interest lies with the individual practitioner, that he/she cannot delegate the decision, and that he/she cannot be required by a superior to disclose or withhold information against his/her will.

(5) That a practitioner who chooses to breach the basic principle of confidentiality in the belief that it is necessary in the public interest must have considered the matter sufficiently to justify that decision.

(6) That deliberate breaches of confidentiality other than with the consent of the patient/client should be exceptional.

Appendix 4

Decisions and/or comments on studies in Chapters 12 and 13

CASE A1

This case study provides a description of a night in a labour ward of a midwifery unit that began very badly and steadily got worse.

There were a number of issues about the context in which the case occurred that caused the members of the committee grave concern. These included (1) the fact that the workload on the night in question was excessive but the response from the immediate managers inadequate; (2) the fact that this midwife had, with colleagues, been instrumental in drawing the pressure of work and low morale in the midwifery unit to the attention of senior management some time before and received no response but had meanwhile noted a press report indicating that the health authority had been told that the unit's staffing was satisfactory; and (3) that the nursing officer and other midwifery sister in the unit had a distorted view of their professional accountability.

This midwife realised fully the significance of her failure on the night in question to see the importance of CTG readings to which, in normal circumstances, she would have reacted at a time and in such a way as to prevent the tragedy that occurred. It was clear to the Committee that she had already learned every lesson that was to be learned from the incident and did not need her peers on the committee to draw those to her attention.

In many respects, though finding misconduct proved, the Committee saw this midwife as a victim of the situation in which she was employed, the inadequacies of which she had drawn to the attention of her managers as the Code of Professional Conduct requires.

Noting the positive statement of the director of midwifery services about the respondent and having confirmed for themselves through their questioning that she was a knowledgeable, highly motivated and competent practitioner, the committee decided that this midwife could safely be left with the right to practise and that no further action needed to be taken against her. It was not even regarded as necessary to speak words of caution or advice in this case. The committee did, however, express their concern about the environment of care and required that a verbatim transcript be sent to the health authority's chairman.

CASE A2

The members of the Professional Conduct Committee wondered why they were sitting hearing a case of this nature since, rather than acting in a manner that might have been regarded as contrary to the interests of the residents the respondent, through his willingness and ability to exercise his judgment, had fully respected and served those interests. He clearly understood that if you exercise judgment you then become accountable for the judgments that you make. He was willing to defend his judgments before a committee of his peers.

The members of the Committee were also astonished that, having trained with the same employing authority, been deemed sufficiently satisfactory for them to put him into a staff nurse post at the completion of training, and then deemed appropriate to manage this holiday, the respondent nurse had been dismissed from employment. It was felt that this would have been an excessive response even if his judgment had proved to be unsound in the circumstances. The members felt that the case said more about the managers of the institution from ward sister upwards than it did about this young and enthusiastic staff nurse. The Committee took the view that the matters which had clearly occurred should not be regarded as misconduct and the case was therefore closed.

CASE A3

The allegations in this case were brought by the senior house officer and his consultant to whom he complained. The latter was not required in evidence as he had no direct knowledge of the events.

In respect of those matters that came down to the question of whether the doctor or the respondent midwife was to be believed, the case study indicates that, having had the opportunity to hear them both in evidence, the Committee did not believe the doctor.

The midwife was still found guilty of misconduct on three charges. Those concerned with the vaginal examination and the administration of Yutopar were regarded as extremely serious in the particular circumstances of the case. The respondent was removed from the register. One of the things that this case illustrates is that you should not give a medication which you know (or ought to know) is contraindicated by the patient's condition, even if it is properly prescribed.

CASE A4

This case, quite apart from the matter which became the subject of a complaint alleging misconduct, provides a particularly bad example of how community psychiatric nursing services are sometimes set up in a quite inappropriate manner, with inadequate resources and unhelpful lines of responsibility.

It is difficult not to feel sympathy for this mature entrant to psychiatric nursing who, after limited and irrelevant experience, was appointed to establish a CPN service.

In order for the facts alleged to be proved the Professional Conduct Committee members had to be satisfied:

(1) that the information passed to another person was 'confidential', *and*
(2) that it had been released without authority or consent, *and*
(3) that the nurse had released it in breach of his position of trust.

After careful deliberation the Committee was satisfied as to points (1) and (2).

In respect of point (3), however, it took the view that the nurse had made careful enquiries and had every reason to believe that the person with whom he was sharing the information could be seen as a long-standing close friend who just happened to have recently become the man's employer, that he had considered the matter carefully before sharing the information, and that it was hardly his fault in the circumstances that the information was subsequently misused. Indeed, the Committee suspected that the friend had known all along and was willing to turn the proverbial blind eye unless/until it emerged that the information was also known to others. The respondent was able to refer back to some personal notes made at the time and retained that indicated the consideration he had given to the matter.

The Committee decided that, rather than act in breach of his position of trust, he had sought to honour it. The charge was therefore not proved and the case closed.

This case provides an opportunity for a word of warning. Allegations of misconduct concerning breaches of confidentiality are rarely made quickly, but more commonly 18 months or more later when any damaging effects become apparent. The normal rule about confidential information is that you do not disclose it. If you decide that the circumstances in which you find yourself constitute one of the rare exceptions to the rule think it through carefully, make a record of your reasons and keep it safe.

(See UKCC document 'Confidentiality'.)

CASE A5

This is a most unusual case. On the one hand the Committee is faced with an admission of quite serious charges. On the other hand it has been told that the managers at the time of the incident had taken no disciplinary action and that the respondent has since been an apparently satisfactory employee.

The new Director of Nursing's wish, having found recorded evidence of the incident and noting that it had never come to the statutory bodies, to have a wider professional view of the matter is quite understandable.

The Committee regarded the matters as misconduct in a professional sense. Having done so it was tempted to postpone judgment for a period, but eventually rejected this view as it had good references in respect of the respondent covering the last 2 years. The members therefore decided not to remove the nurse from the register but to provide some stern words of caution and some appropriate advice.

The members also expressed the hope that close attention had been paid to the setting in which the incident had happened, since the staffing appeared to have been quite inadequate and the use of such words as 'the horsebox' implied that this incident was almost certainly not unique.

CASE A6

The respondent in this case was in serious contravention of the Introduction and clauses 1 and 8 of the Code of Professional Conduct. She had seriously abused her privileged access to the homes and property of an extremely vulnerable client group.

The manner in which she stepped in and out of her professional role, going as a friend to help pack but changing back to 'the nurse' to write misleading notes about the alleged confused state of the patients was regarded by the Committee as particularly nasty and devious. The patients went to different places at different times so the risk of one patient's concern about her linking up with other such concerns was remote.

In spite of the fact that the respondent was said to be skilful and competent and that she formed good relationships with patients and their relatives the Committee felt that the public interest required that she be removed from the register and so ordered.

CASE A7

You were probably tempted to regard this case as fictional. Unfortunately it states things as they happened in this psychiatric unit.

Quite apart from the behaviour of the respondent in the case, there is cause for concern about the limited attention given to this patient during the morning shift, and the inadequacy of the handover report that left the respondent inadequately informed when first encountering the patient.

None of that, however, justified his reactions to the patient's request. There were other staff on duty and it was never argued in the respondent's defence that the unit was short of staff at the time.

The Committee decided to remove this nurse from the register and also to send a transcript of the hearing to the chairman of the health authority as a means of drawing its concerns about the management of the unit to his attention.

CASE A8

The text of the case study indicates that the Committee, having heard and questioned the witnesses, considered the charges of neglect of the patients in the nursing home and failure to provide a suitable environment of care, to be proved and to be misconduct.

In the absence of the opportunity to question and form an assessment of the respondent's character and her view of her conduct and management in retrospect, the Committee members felt that they had no option but to remove her name from the register with immediate effect.

The Committee expressed its concern at the fact that the number of staff available in that particular area for the inspection of a rapidly increasing number of nursing homes was inadequate as a result of which inspections were less frequent than desirable and always with advanced notice. It was agreed that these concerns be drawn to the attention of the registration authority concerned.

CASE A9

The Committee retired for a long time to discuss the case, that fact alone being indicative of the seriousness with which they regarded the offences. In announcing the decision the Chairman of the Committee made that point, and further indicated that they had not been impressed by the allegations made in the course of the defence against the respondent's professional colleagues, claiming that they had behaved inappropriately and acted in something less than professional competence, since such allegations had not in any way been substantiated. The Chairman added that, since on the respondent's instructions her barrister had contested the facts of the case for two days, it was impossible for the Committee to see it (as had been urged upon them) as 'merely an admitted error'.

On behalf of the Committee the Chairman indicated that, even had the situation contained factors that got in the way of delivery of safe care, it expected someone of the educational and professional background concerned to be challenging of such adverse situations and not accepting of them. In the event the Chairman told the respondent that the Committee had been divided on the matter and that the respondent had come extremely close to removal from the register, but that on balance it had been decided not to take that decision but to speak words of caution and counsel. The Chairman emphasised very strongly that the decision not to remove the respondent from the register in no way condoned her conduct in respect of the patient who was placed at risk by her actions.

CASE A10

The Chairman indicated, in giving the Committee's judgment, that to keep and maintain adequate records was both a fundamental feature of health visiting practice and of professional accountability. She added that clause 2 of the UKCC Code of Professional Conduct makes an omission to do something for which you have responsibility just as serious as an act of commission.

However, noting the numerous testimonials concerning her personal and professional qualities, her obvious commitment and innovative practice, and the climate of change and disagreement in which she had been working, the committee decided to take no further action on the misconduct proved against her.

It was noted that she had acknowledged her own shortcomings in record keeping and recognised that she must personally address the issue if she returned to health visiting practice which she was legally able to do.

CASE A11

As indicated in the text, both the standard of evidence and the standard of proof required at Professional Conduct Committee hearings is very high. Indeed, it is the same as that required in criminal courts.

In this case there was clearly conflict of evidence, and the Committee did not take the view that the allegation was proved to them beyond doubt. The charge was therefore found not proved and the case closed.

The members were, however, profoundly disturbed at the picture of the ward which had emerged in evidence, and the fact that those involved in the case and their managers were tolerating in silence things that were clearly intolerable, and required that a transcript of the evidence be sent with an accompanying letter to the health authority chairman.

CASE A12

The text of this case study drew attention to the positive steps taken by the responsible professional manager in respect of the three respondents. It also drew attention to the various points made in mitigation on their behalf and to the concerns which the proven facts had raised in the minds of the Committee.

Before announcing the decision the Chairman stated that the impression to emerge from the case had been that of a conspiracy of silence which was only broken as a result of action taken by newly qualified nurses. This the Committee regarded as courageous, demonstrating their awareness of their professional responsibility as stated in the UKCC's Code of Professional Conduct. The Committee particularly praised the steadfastness of purpose of one witness who, from the time she observed things which caused her grave concern when she was a student, had persisted in her determination to bring those concerns into the open and achieve proper investigation of them in spite of the obstruction she encountered.

After considerable deliberation, and putting in the balance the reprehensible actions or omissions of the three respondents, the things which emerged about them in mitigation, and the subsequent extremely positive enabling work done by their senior manager following his decision not to dismiss them from employment, the Committee decided that no further action should be taken in any of the three cases other than to give some advice as to the respondents' future conduct.

The Chairman, however, reiterated that the misconduct of which the enrolled nurse had been found guilty was grave since she had handled patients inappropriately, abrogated her responsibility of care, and failed to accord respect to the beliefs of a patient, in all of which respects she had contravened the UKCC's expectations of practitioners as set out in the Code of Professional Conduct. As for the ward sister, it was emphasised that a person holding such a post has a responsibility to ensure that the standards of practice on a ward are acceptable, that activities are monitored, and that complaints are appropriately investigated irrespective of the views held about a member of staff about whom complaints were received. In respect of the nursing officer, the Chairman indicated the Committee's view that she was a victim of circumstances who had acted inappropriately when placed in an impossible position by her manager.

CASE A13

Arrangements were quite deliberately made for the Committee to hear expert evidence about the running of specialist units of this type before moving into specific evidence relating to the case. Setting the particular tragic facts of this case against the background provided by the expert witnesses, the Committee were gravely concerned at the blatantly obvious hazards to patients and staff existing in this unit. Their consideration of this led them to the view that the nurse-midwife was as much a victim as the deceased baby.

The Committee decided that in the appalling circumstances of the case and especially the fact that the managers of the unit were aware of the existence of dangerous practices, it would not regard this person as guilty of misconduct. The case was therefore closed.

CASE A14

This case faced the Committee with a serious dilemma. There had been a tragic outcome, though the possibility of this happening without the administration of an excessive quantity of the prescribed antidote must have been a distinct possibility. Here were two experienced, conscientious and effective nurses who had been striving to do their best in extremely difficult circumstances and had (as the Code of Professional Conduct requests) drawn attention to the dangers of their work situation and to the fact that it was a place with an accident waiting to happen. Unfortunately they had received a firm brush-off from their managers.

Having considered the submission by two lawyers on behalf of the respondents, the Committee took the view that the admitted facts would not be regarded as misconduct in view of the appalling context within which the unfortunate incident occurred. The Chairman, on behalf of the Committee, publicly criticised the managers.

CASE A15

The Professional Conduct Committee which heard this case, like its equivalent on many other days, was almost certainly ready to forgive a genuine mistake made under pressure at the end of a busy day. What it could not forgive was the dishonesty with which the mistake was compounded when the matter of the missing instrument came to light.

It seemed to be a case in which pride got in the way of taking an action in the patient's interests.

It should be noted from the text of the case study that, by the time of the hearing, the respondent had obtained a post as a theatre sister, this seemingly being obtained without references being taken up, such a high premium being placed on operating theatre skills.

After very careful consideration the Committee decided to postpone judgment for 3 months (the shortest possible period of postponement) and to require for the resumed hearing a reference from the respondent's new employer which had to be written with knowledge of the facts.

Although it is fairly incidental to this case as it affected the respondent, it is worth recording that the Committee felt that the response of the two night nurses had been less than adequate, although the degree of response from them was probably fairly typical of that which might have been expected from the average registered nurse.

CASE A16

It is obviously preferable for a newly registered nurse to obtain her first experience as a staff nurse on familiar territory. Where this does not prove possible, and particularly where the search for work results in a young person moving a long distance to an unfamiliar setting, it is incumbent on those who employ her to ensure that their introduction to the place and their induction to the work is thorough and comprehensive.

The Committee members were extremely concerned that, in this case, such did not appear to have happened, since as the induction programme was of only 3 days duration, it gave very little opportunity for a thorough orientation to a different setting. In addition, it became clear that, since this respondent was a RSCN and the night sisters were not, she (though newly registered) was led to believe that they regarded her as the expert on paediatrics and there was not a great deal of point in calling upon the night sisters. The Committee members were also concerned at the fact that those who employed her seemed to be expecting her to demonstrate the same degree of knowledge, skill and maturity as they reasonably could from a person of several years standing on the register.

The facts were clearly set out in the case study, and it is indicated that they were admitted. The young woman who appeared with an excellent solicitor did not in any way wish to argue that those facts were not misconduct, and the Committee so found.

At the mitigation stage it emerged that, unlike many others, she had busily occupied her time with further education at a polytechnic to obtain a professional qualification in social work so that, were her registration as a nurse removed, (and she was emphatic that she did not wish that it happen) she was equipped to work in another professional sphere. The Committee respected her greatly for these endeavours, and noted the excellent references she had received in respect of work in an unqualified capacity that she had been doing in both health and social work settings to help fund her further studies.

The members felt that this respondent was very much a victim of the circumstances in which she worked, were satisfied that she had learnt a great deal and grown in insight as a result of her unfortunate experience, and decided that a few words of caution and counsel was quite sufficient.

CASE A17

This was an example of a nurse who was taking advantage of her position and clearly contravening clauses 1 and 8 of the Council's Code of Professional Conduct.

Had the matter not come to light the respondent would have obtained for £140 an antique dining table which would comfortably seat eight, with a set of eight matching antique chairs, and a number of other valuable items which together were of far greater value. Although the patient might have been unusual in respect of those who are the subject of Court of Protection Orders, in that she was still regarded as able to live alone, she was certainly deemed incapable of managing her own financial affairs and it was in this respect that particular advantage was taken of her.

The Committee also particularly disliked the way in which the young community service volunteer, newly moved away from home because of the difficulty of finding work in his own locality, was used first as a means of moving the furniture and of handing over the money, and subsequently that attempts were made to get him to say that the money was a loan from the respondent so that he could buy furniture for his deprived parents. The respondent said that they were apparently in serious need, without carpets and bedding and the like, so an antique table and chairs would not have seemed the thing that they most urgently required.

The decision of the Committee was to remove this lady from the register.

CASE A18

This respondent had been made the subject of a probation order by the Court before which she pleaded guilty. It was therefore not a true conviction for the purposes of the Professional Conduct Committee. The key evidence was that of the police officer.

The Committee was seriously concerned at the major breach of trust which the offences represented. It recognised, however, from the medical reports sent in by the respondent that there had been and remained some serious concern in respect of her health which might possibly have affected her ability to exercise judgment. For this reason the members decided to refer the case for consideration by the Health Committee.

CASE A19

In this case the facts were admitted. The Committee agreed with the respondent that those facts were misconduct. The members were deeply troubled by the respondent's willingness to tolerate what was clearly intolerable and dangerous.

However, given that some nurse managers had taken her into nursing employment with full knowledge of the facts, the committee decided to postpone judgment for six months and to recommend a programme aimed at enhancing her knowledge, increasing her competence and making her more assertive. At the resumed hearing at the end of that period it appeared that the programme had achieved a great deal and the nurse had become a person striving to achieve good standards and with an enquiring approach to practice.

CASE A20

This case study reproduces the statement which the respondent made in writing to the Investigating Committee, and which was also put to the Professional Conduct Committee.

The members felt that the statement superbly illustrated the problems of seeking to deliver good quality nursing care at the present time and irrespective of the speciality. As so often happens in cases from the mental handicap speciality, this caring young woman was herself a victim of the circumstances in which she worked, her vulnerability being made greater by virtue of the fact that she wanted so much to practise well.

The members were particularly aware that had she not told others that she had slapped the resident no-one would have ever known. It was also noted that she was not really able to withdraw from the situation as the policy on violent incidents would have had her do, since to do that would have left the weaker resident at serious risk.

Taking into account all the circumstances, although regarding the slapping of a patient as misconduct, the Committee placed it very low on the spectrum of such offences and took no action. Further to that the members wished this nurse well and expressed the hope that she would soon find employment in caring for the mentally handicapped at which she was clearly very competent. Critical words were addressed to the managers.

CASE A21

As in a substantial percentage of the cases heard by the Committee, the respondent in this case was not the only person with something to answer for. Indeed, it could be argued that she was something of a scapegoat since she was not the senior of the three nurses on duty at the time, and although she was the one who had turned the alarm on the machine off, one of her colleagues had subsequently undertaken the patient's observations and had not turned it on again, and in any event the practice of so doing was well established and engaged in by medical and nursing staff. It rather seemed as if, since a patient had died, the health authority had to have a sacrificial lamb, so this nurse was dismissed from employment and made the subject of allegations of misconduct to the statutory body.

The Committee felt that her actions had been less than satisfactory, but also felt that others not before them and who had not been made the subject of any complaint were as culpable or possibly more culpable.

Given the culpability of others and the previously good record of this nurse who was clearly the wiser for the experience, the Committee, although finding her guilty of misconduct, decided that no further action was needed other than that she be given some words of caution and counsel.

CASE A22

The Committee was appalled that those responsible for the hospital in which this had occurred had rushed into integration of the ward for male and female elderly patients without first satisfying themselves that the ward design was appropriate, and that all the necessary things had been done and clothing, etc., provided to maintain privacy and dignity for the patients.

The case presented something of an enigma, since the sister concerned had apparently maintained excellent standards both before and after the 1 year period when this male nursing assistant (with whom she apparently shared a number of common interests) was placed on her ward. The case was being watched closely by the relations of the elderly and subsequently deceased patient who was the subject of all the charges, they having previously stimulated the health authority concerned to hold a substantial enquiry into the whole affair. The text of the case study makes clear that submissions were upheld in respect of charges (1) and (2) and were rejected in respect of (3), (4) and (5). It also makes it clear that the Committee found the facts in (3), (4) and (5) proved and to be misconduct.

After considerable deliberation the Committee determined to postpone judgment for 1 year and to require that for the resumed hearing one of the references come from a person who had direct-line management responsibility for this respondent.

CASE A23

In deliberating upon this case the Committee was concerned about the evident antipathy which existed between the community unit and the consultant obstetric unit, even though they were communally joined with only an unlocked door between them. Concern was also felt at the fact that this midwife had manifestly failed to sustain and had certainly not improved her professional knowledge and competence. Still further, the Committee was concerned at the fact that having removed this midwife from the list of those who had student attachments because she was inappropriate for the purpose, the midwifery managers of the authority had again placed a student midwife with her after a lapse of time during which they had done nothing to enable her to fulfil a wider role.

The decision of the Committee was to remove this midwife from the professional register.

CASE A24

The members of the Committee found this case profoundly disturbing.

Notwithstanding her long experience as a community midwife and her attendance at a number of regular midwifery refresher courses, this midwife had clearly failed to honour that clause of the Code of Professional Conduct which required her to maintain and improve her professional knowledge and competence.

Her failures were so numerous and her lack of insight in respect of her conduct of the case so great that the Committee felt it had no alternative but to remove her name from the one part of the register on which it had been entered.

CASE A25

A number of things concerned the Committee about this hearing which the respondent did not attend. Anxiety particularly centred around the fact that the night sister did not pursue the matter or arrange for someone else to do so when she failed to receive answers to her telephone calls.

The decision of the Committee was to remove this nurse from the professional register.

STUDY B1

This practice nurse had to decide whether this set of circumstances might possibly be regarded as one of the rare exceptions in which a breach of the important principle of confidentiality could be justified. She realised that such justification must depend on a public interest argument. She decided, on balance, to do nothing but to enjoy spending the money received from the insurance company.

STUDY B2

After some consideration of her limited range of options and being determined to find a genuine solution to the problem rather than an expedient response, the nurse arrived at a decision. Rather than ask her managers what she should do, she declared to them what she was going to do. She indicated that she was personally going to conduct a review of work and working practices in the unit over a period of several weeks, that she would spend time with all members of staff on all wards and all shifts. She provided for her managers the terms of reference she had set herself for the review and stated the date on which she would provide a report complete with decisions and/or recommendations.

That done, she proceeded as she said she would. Her review showed that her cause for concern was well-founded and that the changes she was therefore introducing were necessary in the interests of patients. The foundation of her case was so secure that it could not reasonably be challenged. She appeared to have achieved the change without making the unqualified staff (whose role was substantially changed) feel devalued.

STUDY B3

The events really began when the staff were told of the redeployment plan, but did not ask for confirmation in writing of their assumption, or alternatively for instruction to render them competent for any wards to which they might be directed.

As a first move the nurse refused to go, stating to the night sister that it would be dangerous. She cited in aid clause 4 of the Code of Professional Conduct and was unimpressed by the night sister telling her she must go as there was nobody else to go. The night sister called the night nursing officer to speak to the nurse. She repeated the demand, but supplemented it with some emotional blackmail statements about the poor children in danger. Initially the nurse asked why one of the night sisters was not covering the ward in that case, and repeated her refusal.

After further pressure from her two superiors she said that she would go to the ward, but only after she had sat and written a document stating all the reasons why she felt it to be wrong. She said she would give one copy to the nursing officer, send one to the general manager and keep the third herself for a long time in case there were any long-term repercussions of the events of the night. Then she went. Three hours later there was a rush of emergency admissions and the nurse was recalled to the operating department.

STUDY B4

The nurse in this case felt that she had to be sure of her evidence before raising her concerns with either the surgeon or her manager. However, just as she felt she had sufficient evidence events overtook her, in that she was faced with a patient confident that the outcome of surgery would be what the nurse was sure it would not be.

Her immediate reaction was to tell the patient that her observations over the period she had worked there led her to believe that a radical mastectomy would be performed. The patient was extremely distraught and asked what could be done. The nurse took the unorthodox step of arranging for her to be transferred to a hospital under a different management and to be seen urgently by another surgeon. She did not have a radical mastectomy. The patient was very grateful. The nurse had to face and combat the wrath not only of the surgeon but her managers.

STUDY B5

The young staff nurse in this case was quite clear that the doctor's stated intention was not only illegal and unethical but also impractical.

She told the doctor that she had no intention of cooperating and that she would make a record of the unconsented testing and her reasons for refusing to cooperate.

The doctor decided not to proceed with the blood test.

STUDY B6

This incident raised particular difficulties for someone who had only just returned to nursing after a long career break and to a sphere of practice of which she had no previous experience.

She had no doubt, however, that what she had observed was not acceptable, but lacked confidence to tackle it while still in employment. She resigned her post and then notified the authority with which the home was registered.

STUDY B7

The nurses, having tested their concerns as described, bluntly told the anaesthetists that they knew they had been deceived, and that, while it was for the doctors to prescribe what they wished, they (the nurses) would not administer doses such as those prescribed. Further to that, they would feel it necessary to make a record of their reasons and would contemplate informing the parents of any children for whom such excessive doses were prescribed without consent. There was a sudden return to orthodox prescribing.

STUDY B8

The enrolled nurse quickly decided that she did not require a friend who neglected patients' interests in this way and told her superiors without further delay.

STUDY B9

The nurses in this study were deeply conscious of their undertakings to their clients and the importance of confidentiality.

They indicated that they had no objection to their professional managers having access to their diaries to check on the accuracy of their travel claims, but did not wish to be the means by which some of their clients became inadvertently identified. Their managers agreed to this revised arrangement.

STUDY B10

The nurse in this case was justifiably disturbed by the response and attitude of his immediate manager. He convinced himself that he could not limit his concern to the one person who was his patient at the time but must have concern also for other vulnerable young people who would be in contact with this patient when he was discharged in the near future.

Given his belief that the patient was telling the truth and genuinely wanted to make known his past behaviour in this request, in spite of his manager's comments (which, surprisingly were supported by the psychiatrist), the nurse shared his information with the psychiatric social worker and together they initiated some appropriate action.

STUDY B11

The nurse in this case was faced with an additional difficulty in that, though only a few miles away from the hospital in which she worked in the ITU, the private hospital was located in the territory of the adjacent health authority and was therefore inspected and registered by them. She was convinced that she must raise her concerns in an appropriate manner. Those concerns related to both the frequency with which transfer to the ITU was necessary and to the possibility that unnecessary operations may be occurring. She was convinced that she had an advocate role to perform for future patients. The method she chose is not known.

STUDY B12

The contention of the nursing officer is that to do what the psychiatrists want would be tantamount to unlawful seclusion. It would certainly be an infringement of the freedom of the individual patients concerned. In addition, to comply with the stated requirement was not possible with the staffing levels existing and to even try would greatly reduce the service available to the other patients. In this he was supported by the charge nurses.

He therefore insisted that, if the psychiatrists continued to request that this arrangement should apply, they should prepare a document setting out in detail their reasons and the benefits that they believed would result from it. To this he would add a document stating, on behalf of himself and the clinical nurses, their reasons (of principle and practicability) why this method was considered inappropriate.

Faced with this insistence that reasons for the requirement be stated in writing, the psychiatrists withdrew the instruction.

STUDY B13

The clinical nurse manager in this particular case was being placed in a very difficult position. He was assisted, however, by the fact that two other clinical nurse managers with responsibilities in other specialist areas, having noted his approach to the problem and his reference to the authority's agreed standards, made similar representations. The result was that the senior managers were persuaded to recognise the effects of their financial decisions and to agree to reduce service provision to that which enabled the publicised standards to be met.

STUDY B14

Although the ultimate effect on the patient in this case of withdrawing feeding is the same as that achieved by unplugging the machine where a patient is totally dependent on a ventilator, the time scale to achieve that effect is much greater. A point between the two extremes of removing the tube and thus shortening the time had been rejected. The traumatising effect such a period can have on those whose normal activities are geared to caring cannot simply be dismissed and all staff ordered to comply with the medical instructions.

This is not a situation which is covered by any conscience clause in United Kingdom law. The UKCC's Code of Professional Conduct is not a formula for being selective about which patients a nurse will agree to care for.

The sensitive manager in this case invested a great deal of personal time in providing support for the staff through the period of weeks prior to the patient's death. With difficulty, rotas were organised so that any nurses who felt unable to provide care for the patient or who might feel tempted to break ranks and provide feeding through the nasogastric tube were moved elsewhere or allocated to other patients. No nurse was forced to be party to something they found unacceptable. The period of support for those involved continued well beyond the death of the patient.

STUDY B15

Clause 9 of the Code of Professional Conduct and the supplementary advisory document 'Confidentiality' (see Appendix 3) are relevant to this case. Although emphasising the importance of confidentiality, the latter document states that it is a rule with certain exceptions. Those exceptions focus around a 'public interest' justification.

In this case, after weighing up the risks and benefits on each side, the nurse decided to inform the police.

Table of Cases

Index